RECLAIM YOUR HEALTH

Learn how to overcome the most common chronic illnesses

ALZHEIMER'S DISEASE

By Award Winning Author

DR HARRIS PHILLIP

The contents of this book is for informational purposes only and is not intended to diagnose, treat, cure, or prevent any condition or disease. You understand that this book is not intended as a substitute for consultation with a licensed practitioner. Please consult with your own physician or healthcare specialist regarding the suggestions and recommendations made in this book. The use of this book implies your acceptance of this disclaimer.

Disclaimer

The publisher and authors are not responsible for any specific health needs that may require medical supervision. If you have underlying health problems or have any doubts about the advice contained in this book, please contact a qualified medical doctor or an appropriately trained health care professional. It is not intended as, and should not be relied upon as, medical advice despite having an author with 30+ years' experience in practice in the medical field.

The information contained within this book series, Reclaim Your Health: learn how to overcome the 9 most common chronic health challenges in modern times: Alzheimer's disease is not intended to be used in the place of your general practitioner's advice or your family doctor's advice. This book series is provided for general information only and to empower readers by providing them with relevant information on the disease in an easily digestible format, thus ensuring their visits with their healthcare professional are richer and more rewarding. It will go a long way in helping you understand the pathognomonic features of this commonly seen chronic conditions called Alzheimer's Disease, and it will provide you with some usable tools which you can employ to protect yourself from the daily insults on our bodies.

CONTENTS

Foreword

By Professor Ali Nakash

While continuing with his 30+ years' experience in clinical practice, Harris has decided to sum up much of what he has gained from seeing and treating thousands, maybe millions, of patients with a myriad of medical problems over the years. In his summary, which has been compiled into a series of twelve chunk-sized books, the reader is provided with usable tools which are presented in a simple, readily digestible format to allow everyone to benefit. From the least medically inclined among us, to the nursing student, the pharmacy student, the nurse, the pharmacist, the midwifery student, the midwife, the medical student, and the trained doctor, whether junior or senior. In essence there are useful nuggets of easy-to-follow guidance for all.

In the first book in the series, he starts with a disease we all dread. Many including my wife call it that disease…. You certainly know the disease to which I refer, it is cancer.

Reading through the pages of the first book in this series, I was immediately impressed with the presentation. Such a complex condition was condensed into such simple and easy-to-follow guidance. Not only has he addressed cancer from its cellular level, but he has also extended the discussion to allow you, the reader, to appreciate plausible causative agents for this condition once it is initiated. He gives some insight into how the disease process flourishes, and towards the end of the book he addresses how we can make ourselves cancer-proof.

Making ourselves cancer-proof I find particularly interesting since it allows both medical and non-medical personnel to explore avenues through which they can empower both themselves and their patients as together we fight this dreaded disease.

In the other books of this series which are being completed, the approach is the same, whether it is addressing Alzheimer's disease, cardiovascular disease, diabetes, or the other chronic health challenges of our time. I am particularly impressed with the presentation, the relative simplicity, and the inherent usefulness of this series. This doubtlessly will not only empower, but also serve as a useful companion handbook on our journey to reclaiming our health.

Mr. Phillip is an award-winning author for his book, STOP! It's Not Too Late!: Adding Years to Your Life and Life to Your Years Using the BMS Model, a book which I call an encyclopaedic guide to healthy living. But in this book series I think he has outdone himself as he seeks to provide the tools that we all need to reclaim our health.

He has most definitely put his years of training and experience in capsule form through the various books in this series. Mr Phillip is a trained senior consultant obstetrician and gynaecologist and has displayed his abundance of knowledge through the ease with which he addresses the various chronic health challenges of our times.

This series, for me, represents an interesting and empowering piece of medical science which has been presented in a digestible format for even the non-medical personnel among us. I am therefore moved to make this bold prediction that once you start reading these books, you will find it difficult to stop because of the timeliness and appropriateness of their contents.

Introduction

Several years ago, I was employed as a teacher, which incidentally was my first professional job. While entering the classroom to deliver a biology lecture to a group of students at the Saint Andrews High School, who were preparing to write the General Certificate of Education examination (GCE or GCSE, as referred to in the UK), a young man who claimed he had no interest in Biology collected his books and was leaving the classroom to go to the library, as I entered to deliver the lecture. The lecture was designed to highlight the characteristics of living things and to help distinguish the living from the dead. I commenced the lecture with the statement, 'once one starts living, he/she starts dying'. Inherent in that statement is that both living and dying are processes. Even deeper is the realisation that what we refer to as life is simply a grant of two dates and a dash. Upon hearing this introduction, the young man made an about-turn and asked permission to attend my class. I did not convert him into a biologist, but he left the class much better informed. Today that young man is a politician. We are granted a date of birth and a date of death: between these two dates is the dash and that is the focus of this book, how can we extend the dash to delay our date of death. I prefer to look at the whole scenario as a rubber band that can be stretched between two points, the two points being the date of birth and the date of death. We can do nothing about our date of birth, that date is beyond our control, but if my analogy of a rubber band is fully understood, and since our date of birth cannot be seriously influenced by our action or inaction, for the rubber band concept to hold, it means that the dash can be extended and thus we can delay our date of death.

My paternal grandmother, for instance, lived to a ripe old age of 115 years. She lived a fully independent life, still being able to cook and care for herself in her 115th year. This is not widespread, I hear you say, and my response is why not? Do we have any skills, knowledge, or abilities in the current era to approach this lifespan and make it more of the expected norm as opposed to an occasional event?

It is with this burning desire that I have used my medical knowledge, gleaned in the field, as well as my extensive research, the skills of which I learned as a university student in organic and biochemistry at a top 10USA university as I pursed a PhD degree in Biochemistry. This training not only provided me with the skills and tools which I needed to pursue the more inquisitive aspect of my person, but also has alerted me to the value of research. Thus, when faced with a challenging question, I revert to research to help me determine the answer.

In observing the lifestyle of my paternal grandmother, my 30+ years of medical practice, drawing on the knowledge gleaned through my research, and from my study in organic chemistry, leading to my Master's degree and my sojourn through the biochemistry classroom, I believe that we have an opportunity to delay the second date, the date of death, by stretching in rubber band style the duration of the dash. This is therefore the purpose of this book: providing tools, suggestions and basic information which will hopefully allow you to prolong your dash and live a more dynamic and healthier lifestyle, thus adding years to your life and life to your years.

I will aim to provide sections on each of the nine most common chronic ailments of our time, suggesting how best one can delay the effect of the insult on our bodies, hence allowing us to live a more complete, fun-filled life, a guide to which has been developed in one of my earlier books, about using the BMS approach, an award-winning book.

In this book series we will look at cancer, Alzheimer's, dementia and diseases of the brain, heart disease and strokes, diabetes, arthritis, obesity, chronic lung diseases, and chronic kidney diseases, hoping that this serves as a useful handbook – guide, if you will – in understanding and defeating the most common chronic ailments affecting human beings on planet earth.

I know that you may be stunned: why has a trained obstetrician and gynaecologist got involved in the writing of books addressing various aspects of health, some of which may be remote from obstetrics (care of pregnant ladies during their pregnancy and childbirth and for the first42 days after ending the pregnancy) and gynaecology (the branch of medicine which deals with the functions and diseases specific to women and girls, specifically those relating to the reproductive system)? To this my response is simple:

It is the only medical discipline which allows one to practise all the facets of medicine. It therefore means that any good obstetrician and gynaecologist, because of the demands on his scope of practice, needs to be above average in his knowledge of internal medicine, surgery, paediatrics, social and preventative medicine, care of the elderly, and neonatology. Hence my familiarity with these various disciplines and the related physiology has empowered me in the provision of this book series which I am hopeful will be an empowering tool to help many understand elements of their health, while simultaneously allowing them to know when things are wrong and therefore see the need to seek medical advice. Hopefully the message is that the earlier a disease process is found, the more options will be available for management and the more likely a full cure will be realised.

BOOK 2
ALZHEIMER'S DISEASE

CHAPTER 1
Alzheimer's, Dementia and Brain Health

- The brain

- Threats to brain health

- Memory

- Short-term memory

- Long-term memory

- The biology of memory loss

- Identifying memory decline

- Memory enhancers

- Are there any tools available to us to enhance our memory?
  - Alpha -GPC
  - Huperzine A
  - Bacopa monnieri
  - Lion's mane
  - Ginkgo Biloba

- Pause For Thought.

- Take Home Nuggets

- Pages for personal notes

Have you ever wondered why the brain is at the upper extremity of most animals, and the direction of the animal's movement is in the direction of the brain? Could this reflect the intended role of the brain as the master organ, designed to direct the activity of the organism on which it was fitted? Needless to claim that the brain is a complex master organ that directs the myriad of activities directly or indirectly, consciously or subconsciously, that go into keeping us alive and guiding us to become the beings into whom we merge.

It is necessary to maintain this exceptional organ in its best state of health. Unfortunately, this does not always occur. We repeatedly see the decline of this organ with time. The triggers, though, almost always environmental, are varied.

Threats to brain health

We recognise the brain: a soft, mushy structure housed, and some may say protected, in a hard, bony box, the skull; but not only is the skull protective, it can also be a source of injury to the brain with adverse potential sequelae. We learn of contrecoup injuries, which involve a contusion on the opposite side to the actual site of impact to the head, a phenomenon commonly seen among boxers. After years of trauma to their heads we see a slurring of their speech, jerkiness of their movements, a sort of Parkinsonian-type effect, as was evidenced in Mohammad Ali before his death. The injury may cause immediate transformation or may follow a prolonged, tortuous path. In this scenario there is usually an obvious predisposing event, but in others there is a less clearly visible causation that insidiously negatively affects memory and powers of recall, a phenomenon called dementia, or a decline in mental ability severe enough to interfere with daily life.

These injuries, which may be macroscopic, can lead to compression- type injuries, which may present with headaches, visual disturbances or even death, since the skull cannot expand. Brain swelling can lead to a herniation of the brain into the spinal column, a fatal event.

The purpose of this chapter is the exploration of a variety of avenues which are useful in protecting us from damaging our brains, and thus preventing the sequelae from a damaged brain.

Memory

Among the most easily visible pointers of the functionality of the brain, I am sure you will agree, is memory. The scientist tells us that there are two major types of memory: short-term memory and long-term memory.

Short-term memory: It is defined as the capacity for holding a small amount of information in an active, readily available state for a short interval. The duration of short-term memory is estimated to be a few seconds, for example the type of memory used to recall a telephone number that has just been recited to you.

Long-term memory: This type of memory process takes information from the short-term memory store and creates long-lasting memories. The duration of these memories varies in time from a few hours earlier to several years or decades earlier.

For ease of recall, long-term memory is subdivided into three types: memory associated with how to do procedures would be different from other types of long-term memory; so to distinguish this type, one talks of **procedural long-term memory** which relates to implicit long-term memory responsible for knowing how to do things, that is essentially, memory of motor skills. For example, once you start walking, you don't have to try to remember that to move, one foot must move first and it is the followed by the movement of the second foot. There is also **semantic memory**, which relates to long-term memory responsible for storing information about the world. For example, you will know who is the President of the USA. Finally, there is **episodic memory**: this is the type of long-term memory that involves conscious recollection of previous experiences together with their context in terms of time, place and associated emotions. A part of the brain called the hippocampus is critically involved in forming these episodic memories. Examples of episodic memories include information on where you placed your keys, and memories of a holiday you have had.

Memory is but a tiny part of brain functioning. According to Johns Hopkins neurologist, Barry Gordon, five of his top suggestions for protecting brain health are:

(1) We need to engage our hearts daily by employing heart-pumping exercises. It is no secret that exercise is beneficial in lowering one's risk of hypertension and diabetes, and it improves mood as well as sleep. Needless to advise on the role of aerobic exercise in weight control. Of

great value is that the benefits add up no matter at what age you choose to start your aerobic exercises.

(2) Medical problems can also have a deleterious effect on brain health. Medical problems such as diabetes – in fact, Alzheimer's is considered by some to be type 3 diabetes. Strokes, heart disease and hypertension are also known to damage brain health. The insult on the brain's health can be less impactful by reducing your risk for these conditions or by controlling them.

(3) Adequate amount of sleep is also integral to ensuring brain health. There is increasing evidence that sleep disorders can have a negative influence on mental function. Two common sleep robbers are obstructive sleep apnoea and stress.

(4) Drugs used to treat anxiety, such as sedatives, can affect memory adversely.

(5) Keeping your brain active by challenging it through learning new things can prove beneficial. Pursuing interest that keeps you connected with others may be better for brain health. Having a conversation with a friend over lunch, for example, may be a better contributor to brain health than memorising numbers in reverse.

The biology of memory loss

Researchers have told us that the substance necessary for keeping our minds sharp is a neurotransmitter called acetylcholine. Younger minds are able to store large quantities of information. This is rendered possible by the neurotransmitter acetylcholine, which maintains and strengthens neural connections which are integral to having a sharp memory. With increasing age, though, the levels of acetylcholine decline and with this comes the weakening of the neural pathways required to retrieve information.

Interestingly, increasing levels of acetylcholine create new neural connections, which enhance the information-sharing network of your mind. This process restores retentive memory, clears focus, and encourages confident decision-making.

Identifying memory decline

There are telltale signs which are associated with memory decline, and for simplicity they are divided into three stages. Stage 1: Senior moments. Here common memory lapses become more frequent. The ease with which you misplace everyday items or difficulty in recall of words increases in frequency. Stage 2: Brain fog. Learning new concepts becomes increasingly difficult; one finds the ability to recall information increasingly difficult. There is difficulty concentrating on the task at hand, or you tend to feel overwhelmed when multiple issues demand your attention. Stage 3: Social withdrawal. Difficulty with one's memory becomes increasingly obvious to those around you. Names, dates and facts slip from your mind more easily. There is an increased tendency to repeat yourself and you may visibly struggle to follow long stories. So, social withdrawal, even from friends and family, seems a coping mechanism to avoid embarrassment.

Memory enhancers

We accept a gradual decline in our memory as a natural consequence of aging or getting older. Recent studies indicate that this begins to occur in the early to mid-forties. To store and retrieve new information, the brain relies on acetylcholine, which plays an essential role in forming neural connections. Unfortunately, this neural transmitter, acetylcholine, decreases as we get older, limiting our ability to create new short-term memories. This may explain the difficulty we experience as we get older in creating short-term memories. We may find it easier to recall people or events from decades earlier, but may struggle to remember where we placed our car keys.

Are there any tools available to us to enhance our memory?

No one can stop the impact of time on our memory, but supplements and a healthy lifestyle can help in keeping your mind sharp and keeping you focussed. The combination of supplements and a healthy lifestyle can also help with our concentration and with mental clarity.

Understanding the biology of memory decline and knowing the mechanism by which this can be halted, and even reversed, give us an opportunity to access the memory enhancers on the market and to search for key components that should be present to ensure their efficacy. The focus on these components is based on their ability or inability to boost acetylcholine. The top five natural agents with the proven ability to boost acetylcholine levels based on double-blinded, placebo-controlled trials, the most robust scientific research, are:

(1) **Alpha-GPC:** This is a natural compound found in the brain that transports choline efficiently across the blood-brain barrier and serves as a biological precursor for acetylcholine. In studies it has been shown that supplementation with alpha-GPC can increase the amount of bioavailable acetylcholine for up to 30 hours which results in your brain's ability to make new neural connections and store information efficiently.

(2) **Huperzine A:** This is a compound derived from the Huperzia serrata firmoss, native to India and Southeast Asia. This drug, which is known to enhance memory, brings about its effect by suppressing the action of acetylcholinesterase, the enzyme which breaks down acetylcholine, the neurotransmitter. In 2006 in a study it was shown that daily use of huperzine A markedly increased levels of acetylcholine and significantly improved short-term memory.

(3) **Bacopa monnieri:** also known as brahmi, it is a perennial herb frequently used in traditional ayurvedic medicine for its memory- enhancing properties. It is believed to work in a similar manner to huperzine A by inhibiting the breakdown of acetylcholine in the brain. Studies over a decade ago showed that this herb significantly improved learning and memory retention over placebo.

(4) **Lion's mane:** This ancient Chinese medicinal mushroom has been shown to cross the blood-brain barrier and increase levels of acetylcholine by enhancing the activity of choline acetyltransferase, the enzyme that produces acetylcholine. In 2009, a study indicated that lion's mane increased memory scores without adverse side effects; and

(5) **Ginkgo biloba:** this is derived from the ginkgo tree that is native to China and has been cultivated for many years for its memory- enhancing properties. A 2000 study revealed that ginkgo increases uptake of acetylcholine in the hippocampus. When paired with Bacopa monnieri it brings about a noticeable improvement in memory.

Approximately 40% of people will struggle with age-related memory lapses during their lifetime as one gets older and is common after the age of 65. Hence there is an ongoing public demand for memory-enhancement products.

There are many ineffective supplements with questionable ingredients with no proof of efficacy on the market. The ingredients in most memory boosters can provide noticeable improvements within 30 days. Optimal acetylcholine production leads to maximisation of the brain's ability to create new neural pathways.

Researchers tell us that 3 months of daily use help significantly increase the likelihood of lasting improvement. A patient on effective supplements after the first month will tend to be less forgetful and more focussed.

After the second month, his/her short-term memory gets sharper with greater capacity and faster recall. By month 3 peak improvement in memory is noted: there is greatly improved concentration and alertness. Your confidence in your memory rises.

Pause For Thought

- Why do most organism natural move is in the direction of their heads?

- How is the skull able to cause brain injury?

- What are the types of memory?

- What is our brain's neurotransmitter and how does it work?

- What causes memory decline?

- Can exercise help to protect brain health?

- Are there any useful memory enhancers available?

- How long does it take good memory enhancers to bring about an improvement in memory?

Take Home Nuggets

- The brain is the master organ of the body, we can't live without the brain and the heart.

- Although the skull is protective, under certain conditions it can injure the brain.

- With contact sports there are brain injuries which are lumped together and called traumatic brain injuries (TBI), these can present immediately or can have a devastating effect on a person as they age.

- We can remain sharp and focused because of neurotransmitters which pass information between nerve cells, through synapses. One such neurotransmitter is acetyl choline.

- Though Alzheimer's is a single disease which is continuous, it is conveniently divided into stages.

- There are several suggestions by which one can improve their brain health. These include exercise, proper and effective management of some diseases such as diabetes and high blood pressure.

- Memory can be divided into several different types. The two major divisions are short term memory and long-term memory.

Notes

_____

_____

_____

_____

_____

_____

_____

_____

_____

_____

_____

_____

_____

_____

_____

_____

_____

_____

_____

Notes

_____

_____

_____

_____

_____

_____

_____

_____

_____

_____

_____

_____

_____

_____

_____

_____

_____

_____

_____

Chapter 2
Alzheimer's Versus Dementia: Is There Any Difference?

- Alzheimer's disease
- Incidence of Alzheimer's disease
- Signs and symptoms of Alzheimer's disease
- Does Alzheimer's affect one's lifespan?
- Stages of Alzheimer's Alzheimer's disease
  - Stage 1
  - Stage 2
  - Stage 3
  - Stage 4
  - Stage 5
  - Stage 6
  - Stage 7
- Pause For Thought
- Take Home Nuggets
- Pages for personal notes

Alzheimer's disease is a brain disorder that slowly destroys memory, the thought-process and eventually the ability to carry out the simplest tasks. In people with the late-onset disease type, the symptoms first appear in their mid-sixties. In the early onset variety, it affects persons in the age range between 30 and 65; this type is rare.

Alzheimer's disease was first identified and named after Dr Alois Alzheimer in 1906. This discovery was prompted by the post-mortem findings in the brain tissue of a woman who died of an (until then) unusual mental illness. Her symptoms included memory loss, language difficulties and unpredictable behaviour. The post-mortem examination of her brain revealed findings of abnormal plaques, now referred to as amyloid plaques and tangled bundles of fibres, now referred to as neurofibrillary or tau tangles.

These plaques and tangles in the brain are still considered pathognomonic features of Alzheimer's disease. Another feature found was the loss of connections between different parts of the brain, and from the brain to muscles and organs in the body. There are many other complex brain changes thought to play a role in Alzheimer's disease.

The initial focus of damage is around the areas of the brain involved in memory. It is therefore not surprising that the early signs and symptoms of the disease process are associated with memory dysfunction. The areas of insults include the entorhinal cortex and hippocampus which are the parts of the brain that are essential in forming memories. This later affects areas in the cerebral cortex, such as those areas responsible for language, reasoning and social behaviour. This progresses to other areas of the brain. This progression of the disease process on the brain helps one to understand the progressive symptoms seen in the individuals suffering with the disease.

Incidence of Alzheimer's disease

It is estimated that more than 6 million Americans over age 65 may have Alzheimer's disease; several individuals under age 65 also suffer from this disease process. So, it is evident that unless Alzheimer's can be effectively treated or prevented, the number of cases will continue to increase, since increasing age is the most important known risk factor for Alzheimer's disease.

Signs and symptoms of Alzheimer's disease

Memory problems are among the first signs of Alzheimer's, though the symptoms are person-dependent. That is, in one person the initial symptoms may differ from those in another. Changes in the brain may begin ten years or more before the first symptoms appear. During this very early stage of Alzheimer's, toxic changes are taking place in the brain, including abnormal build-ups of proteins that form amyloid plaques and tau tangles. Previously healthy neurons stop functioning, lose connections with other neurons, and die. There may be many other complex brain changes which play a role in Alzheimer's. As more neurons die, additional parts of the brain are affected, die and the brain begins to shrink. In the final stages of Alzheimer's, damage is widespread and brain tissue has shrunk significantly. Since death is defined in terms of the absence of brain activity, we can easily understand why Alzheimer's is such a devastating disease. It is a gradual death. There may be a decline in finding the right words to express oneself, issues with vision and spatial orientation, faulty reasoning and/or judgement: all form part of the initial presentation of the disease process. Though some older adults may have some memory or thinking problems, called mild cognitive impairment, which can be an early sign of Alzheimer's, not everyone with mild cognitive impairment will develop Alzheimer's disease.

Alzheimer's is a very devastating disease, not only for the afflicted party, but also for those caring for them. These individuals have trouble doing everyday activities like driving, cooking, or even paying bills. Conversing with them may be challenging as they tend to ask the same questions repeatedly, they get lost easily, lose items easily and tend to place these items in odd places, and they seem to get confused with simple things. As the disease progresses, some afflicted persons may become worried, angry or even violent.

Does Alzheimer's affect one's lifespan?

This disease is currently ranked as the seventh leading cause of death in the United States. The leading cause of death in the UK in 2018 was dementia and Alzheimer's disease, accounting for 12.7% of all deaths registered. This disease is therefore sufficiently important to try to arrest its progress, and as indicated above it is also a painful experience to carers as they observe their clients continued decline with no known tools available to cure or halt the decline. Hopefully with this holistic approach we will be able to address this process and bring about a dent in the ravages of this disease.

We find that the time which elapses between diagnosis and death varies from as little as three or four years, if the person is older than 80 years, to as long as 10 or more years, if the person is younger.

Stages of Alzheimer's disease

Though Alzheimer's is a single disease, it has been broken down into seven stages for easy understanding.

Stage 1: Before overt symptoms appear. In this stage, there are changes related to Alzheimer's that begin before symptoms are noticeable. This is often referred to as pre-clinical Alzheimer's disease. It likely begins 10 to 15 years before people have symptoms.

Stage 2: Basic forgetfulness: In this relatively early stage of the disease, Alzheimer's can look like normal-aged forgetfulness. There will be memory lapses, including forgetting people's names or where they have left items or even parked their car. They are still able to drive, perform their daily tasks, work profitably and be social. However, these memory gaps increase in frequency.

Stage 3: Noticeable memory difficulties. Here the memory difficulties become increasingly evident and harder to blame advancing age as purely the cause. It is usually at this stage that the patient is diagnosed. Common difficulties at this stage go beyond forgetting names and misplacing objects. The patient may have trouble remembering recently read materials such as books or magazines; remembering plans and organising becomes increasingly difficult. In addition to having increasing difficulty retrieving a name or word, they have challenges in social settings or at work. It is at this stage that anxiety levels among carers and family begin to rise; with some in denial. These are normal reactions, and the advice would be to speak to your doctor about the observed changes.

Stage 4: Involves continued worsening of the condition and now involves more than memory loss. This may involve difficulty with language, organisation, and calculations. This stage can last for several years in which there will be worsening memory difficulties. The memory of distant past events will be significantly better than their day-to-day memory of more recent events.

Other challenges may involve confusion about the day of the week, and increased risk of wandering off and getting lost. There may be changes in their sleeping pattern, such as restlessness in the night but sleeping during the day. Additionally, there may be appropriate dressing concerns, that is wearing weather-appropriate attire. Social gatherings may become frustrating, and the patient may feel moody or withdrawn. There may be other personality changes such as suspiciousness of others and depression.

Stage 5: In this stage the patient begins to become less independent. They may have difficulty remembering people who are important to them, such as family and friends. Added to this may be emotional changes such as paranoia they may begin hallucinating and having delusions.

Stage 6: Severe symptoms: Here the symptoms are more significant and negatively impact their ability to manage their own care. Communications may also be challenging at this stage; words and phrases can still be used, expression may be difficult, and they may be unable to describe where pain is felt, if they are in pain. It must be understood that these changes are not always present.

Stage 7: Lack of physical control: Alzheimer's disease is a process in which brain cells are progressively destroyed, leading to severe mental and physical impairment.

Pause For Thought

- Is Alzheimer's disease the same as Dementia?
- Was Alzheimer's disease the leading cause of death in the UK in 2018?
- Does Alzheimer's disease affect one's life span?
- Does Alzheimer's disease affect one's short term or long-term memory in its earliest stages?
- Does Alzheimer's disease occur in stages or is it a continuous, progressive disease?

Take Home Nuggets

- Alzheimer's disease is the most common type of Dementia. Alzheimer's is always dementia but dementia is not always Alzheimer's disease.
- Alzheimer's disease shortens one's life span and is a progressive process as parts of the brain progressively dies and shrinks.
- Though Alzheimer's disease is a single disease, it has been broken up into a number of stages so that it can be studied easier.

- Alzheimer's disease may be first suspected in its earlier stages by increased forgetfulness but this will evolve into being lost in familiar surroundings and emotional changes as well as loss of independence.

Notes

Notes

_____

_____

_____

_____

_____

_____

_____

_____

_____

_____

_____

_____

_____

_____

_____

_____

_____

_____

_____

_____

Chapter 3
Dementia

- Dementia

- Signs and symptoms of dementia

- Signs of dementia

- Factors increasing the risk of dementia

- Types of dementia

- Are mental health issues associated with dementia?

- Pause for thought

- Take home nuggets

- Pages for personal notes

Dementia is not a specific disease but rather a general term for impaired ability to remember, think or make decisions that is necessary for everyday activities. Alzheimer's is the most common type of dementia. Although dementia affects older adults, it is not considered to be a part of normal aging.

Signs and symptoms of dementia

The symptoms of this assembly of diseases vary widely from person to person. They have problems with memory, attention, communication, reasoning, judgement, and problem-solving; their visual perception may also be impaired beyond that expected by age-related peers.

Signs of dementia

This may include getting lost in a familiar neighbourhood, referring to familiar objects using unusual words, forgetting the name of a close family member or friend, forgetting old memories, and an inability to complete tasks independently.

Factors increasing the risk of dementia

(1) Age: This is the strongest known risk factor for dementia. Most cases occur at age 65 or older.

(2) Family history: If you have had parents or siblings with dementia, you would be at increased risk.

(3) Race/ethnicity: older negroes are twice more likely to have dementia than whites. Hispanics are about 1.5 times more likely to suffer from dementia than whites.

(4) Poor heart health: high blood pressure, high cholesterol and smoking increase the risk of dementia if not properly treated. Note that the Food and Drug Administration in the USA indicates that some people have developed memory loss or confusion while taking statins (drugs used to lower one's cholesterol). Interestingly, these side effects disappear once the medication is stopped. A pooled analysis of 36 studies found that statins were associated with a decreased risk of dementia.

(5) Traumatic brain injury: Head injuries can increase the risk of dementia, particularly if the head injury is severe or ongoing.

Types of dementia

As stated above, Alzheimer's disease is the most common type of dementia but there are other types of dementia. Among them are:

(a) Vascular dementia, with about 10% of dementia cases linked to strokes or other issues with blood flow to the brain. Diabetes, high blood pressure and high cholesterol are also risk factors. The symptoms will vary depending on the area and size of the brain impacted. The condition gets progressively worse as the number of strokes or ministrokes increases.

(b) There is also Lewy body dementia: In this type of dementia, in addition to memory loss, affected individuals may have movement or balance problems like stiffness or trembling. Affected individuals may also experience changes in alertness, including daytime sleepiness, confusion or staring spells. They may also experience visual hallucinations.

(c) Frontotemporal dementia: This type of dementia most often leads to changes in personality and behaviour. These patients may embarrass themselves or behave inappropriately. There may also be issues with language skills like speaking or understanding.

(d) Mixed dementia. In people of advanced years, aged 80 and older, it is likely to have more than one type of dementia present at the same time. In these cases, disease progression may be faster than if there was only one type of dementia present. And finally:

(e) Reversible causes, such as side effect of medication, increased intracranial pressure, vitamin deficiency and thyroid hormone imbalance.

Are mental health issues associated with dementia?

A recent large new study finds an association between mental health conditions and dementia later in life. While a causal link is yet to be established, mental health issues remain a predictor of dementia. It therefore stands to reason that successfully addressing mental health conditions may help to reduce the likelihood of dementia for older adults.

Pause For Thought

- Is Dementia always the same as Alzheimer's disease?
- Are there any signs and or symptoms of Dementia?
- Are there any risk factors which increases your chance of developing Dementia?
- What are the types of Dementia?
- Are mental health issues associated with Dementia?

Take Home Nuggets

- Dementia is not always Alzheimer's disease. Alzheimer's is the commonest type of dementia.

- The signs and symptoms of Alzheimer's disease are like that for other types of dementia.

- There are various factors which increases one's risk of developing dementia. Old age is a major risk factor.

- There are various types of Dementia, these types are classified based on their causation, the location of the brain that is insulted and they may present differently, still forgetful but they may involve for example personality changes.

- Recently there has been much talk about mental health issues, it is now realised that mental health issues may be related to the development of dementia.

Notes

_____

_____

_____

_____

_____

_____

_____

_____

_____

_____

_____

_____

_____

_____

_____

_____

_____

_____

_____

_____

Notes

_____

_____

_____

_____

_____

_____

_____

_____

_____

_____

_____

_____

_____

_____

_____

_____

_____

_____

_____

_____

_____

_____

_____

Chapter 4
Individualised Combination Therapy (ICT) in Reversing and Even Curing Alzheimer's Disease

- Can Alzheimer's disease be cured?
- Patient 1
- Patient 2
- Patient 3
- Making the ICT protocol person specific
- An in-depth look at the ICT protocol for reversing Alzheimer's disease
- The ICT ten simple steps
  - Step1
  - Other treatments
  - Step 2
  - Treatment
  - Treatment: stress reduction
  - Supplemental treatment
  - Step 3
  - Treatment
  - Supplemental treatments

- o Step 4
- o Treatment
- o Treatment supplements
- o Step5
- o Treatment
- o Step6
- o Step7
- o Treatment
- o Step8
- o Treatment: mental exercise
- o Treatment: physical exercise
- o Step 9
- o Treatment
- o Step10
- o Treatment
- Pause For Thought.
- Take Home Nuggets
- Pages for personal notes

Traditional medicine has led us to believe that Alzheimer's disease is without cure, and once the diagnosis is made there is nothing that we can do to arrest the progress of the disease. This is devastating news for a relative or carer of an individual who has been afflicted. In this book series where I endeavour to take a more holistic approach to addressing the nine most common chronic ailments affecting mankind, I hope to provide you with a combination approach of both non-pharmaceutical and traditional approaches to arrest, reverse and even cure this ailment.

I will give the results from three patients who religiously followed the individualised combination therapy (ICT) protocol in their fight against Alzheimer's disease.

Patient 1: Let us call her Mary. Mary was a 67-year-old who was experiencing increased memory loss over a two-year period. Her job included an extensive degree of travel. It was demanding and highly technical and involved preparation of documents and reports. It became obvious to her employers that she was struggling in the preparation of reports and her analysis of data left a lot to be desired. She was coming to the realisation that she was no longer able to function efficiently on the job and was considering leaving the job. She often got lost driving along familiar roads. It progressed to being unable to find the light switches in her own home and confused about the names of her pets.

Interestingly, her mother had suffered a severe decline in her memory in her early sixties. At the time of her death, she suffered from severe dementia and she spent many years in a nursing home.

Mary began the protocol, and, although she could follow all of the steps (that is she was not in the more advanced stage of Alzheimer's disease, she still experienced a great improvement in her symptoms. Her memory improved dramatically, and she no longer got lost easily. So marked was her improvement that she continued full-time on the job for an additional two and a half years until she was 70 years of age.

As if through a natural experiment, during the protocol the patient developed a viral illness and had to stop the programme. Almost immediately, her memory started to decline but on resuming the protocol, the symptoms disappeared.

The parts of the protocol she completed involved:

- Eliminating simple carbohydrates from her diet.
- Weight loss of 20 pounds.
- Processed food and gluten were eliminated from her diet.
- She increased her intake of fruits, vegetables and wild fish.
- She began studying yoga.
- She meditated for 20 minutes two times per day.
- She used melatonin to help her sleep better.
- She increased the amount of sleep she had to 7–8 hours per night.
- She took 1mg of methylcobalamin each day.
- She used vitamin D3 supplements.
- She used 2000mg of fish oil tablets every day.
- She took 200mg of coenzyme Q10 daily.
- She started using an electric toothbrush and flosser.
- She resumed hormone replacement therapy.
- She fasted for 12 hours between dinner and breakfast.
- She consumed her evening meal at least three hours before bedtime.

- She also committed to a minimum of 30 minutes of exercise for 4–6 days each week.

Patient 2, we will call Mark. Mark was a 69-year-old professional who had been having worsening memory loss over the previous 11 years. In the last two years, the memory loss was progressing at a faster rate. A brain scan in 2003 revealed typical patterns of Alzheimer's disease.

Within 6 months of starting the protocol, Mark had improved and he was now able to remember his daily schedule and people's faces. He was again functional at work. His rapid rate of decline had been arrested.

The protocol used involved:

- Having nothing to eat or drink for at least 3 hours before bed.
- Fasting for 12 hours between dinner and breakfast.
- Eliminating simple carbohydrates and processed foods from his diet.
- Increased consumption of fruit, vegetables, wild fish, grass-fed beef, and organic chicken.
- He took probiotics.
- He took one tablespoon of coconut oil twice daily.
- He increased exercise to swimming 3–4 times a week.
- He took melatonin to help him sleep.
- He increased his sleep to 8 hours per night.
- He took 250mg of Bacopa, 500mg of ashwagandha and 400mg of turmeric each day.

- He took 1mg of methylcobalamin, 0.8mg of methyltetrahydro-folate and 50mg of pyridoxal-5 phosphate daily.

- He took 500mg of citicoline twice-daily.

- He took vitamin C, vitamin D3 and vitamin E each day.

- He took 200mg of coenzyme Q10 daily.

- Mark also took Zinc picolinate 50mg daily.

- He also took DHA and EPA.

Patient 3, we call Debra. Debra was a 55-year-old attorney who had suffered progressive memory loss over a 4-year period. Her children noticed that she would occasionally forget what she was talking about mid-sentence, and her response time was increasing. She spent five months following the protocol and made a tremendous improvement. She was then able to return to work and even pursue further study.

Her protocol treatment included the following:

- Having nothing to eat or drink for at least 3 hours before bed.

- Fasting for 12 hours between dinner and breakfast.

- Eliminating simple carbohydrates and processed foods from her diet.

- Increase her intake of fruits, vegetables and wild fish.

- Exercise 4–5 times per week.

- She took melatonin to help her sleep.

- She tried to get at least 8 hours of sleep nightly.

- She used meditation and relaxation techniques to reduce stress.

- She took 1mg of methylcobalamin 4 times per week.

- She used 20mg of pyridoxine 5'-phosphate per day.

- She used 200mg of citicoline each day.

- She used vitamin D3 supplements.

- 200mg of coenzyme Q10 daily.

- DHA and EPA.

- Used her hormone replacement.

- She reduced her bupropion prescription.

Making the ICT protocol person-specific

The steps in the ICT protocol include diet, exercise for your body and brain, correction of hormonal levels, improving antioxidant levels and gut flora, improving dental hygiene, and adequate sleep.

As shown in the cases above, stopping the protocol can result in a decline in memory to its pre-treatment state, yet on resumption of the protocol, the trend can be reversed. The key features in this protocol revolve around changing one's diet, and managing your vitamins and hormone levels.

An in-depth look at the ICT protocol for reversing Alzheimer's disease

This protocol is an all-natural, at home treatment called the Individualised Combination Therapy, which is tailored to the person suffering with Alzheimer's disease.

This protocol is designed to target multiple known causative factors in the development of Alzheimer's, and not simply on one potential factor. Patients are allowed to undergo multiple clinical tests, inclusive of blood studies, to determine what deficiencies and imbalances exist.

Thus far, 36 deficiencies have been identified; inflammation and hormonal imbalances all play a part in decreasing memory function. To many involved in Alzheimer's research, each deficiency seems to fit together and contribute to the issues with memory evident in Alzheimer's disease. Some people, for example, may have a larger deficit in vitamin D and a smaller deficit in oestrogen, but together these deficits work synergistically to bring about a decline in memory.

The ICT 10 simple steps

For the ICT protocol to be successful, the participant must follow each stage step by step: completing the steps out of order won't necessarily lead to the same results.

Step 1: Reduce inflammation and stabilise blood sugar levels. Alzheimer's disease is often referred to as type 3 diabetes, because of the insulin resistance in the brain. Brown Medical School researchers have been able to show that insulin is produced in both the pancreas and the brain. This explains why individuals suffering from type 2 diabetes are at increased risk of developing Alzheimer's disease. To address this, it is suggested that a diet low in grains, simple carbohydrates and sugars on the low- glycaemic index are recommended.

Instead of processed foods, one should consume plenty of fresh foods, including vegetables and quality meats and fish.

One should avoid eating less than 3 hours from bedtime. A fasting period of at least 12 hours should be allowed between dinner and breakfast daily. Treatment supplements: Recommended supplements for this step are DHA (docosahexaenoic acid, an omega-3 fatty acid), EPA (eicosapentaenoic acid, also an omega-3 fatty acid), and curcumin. Both DHA and EPA reduce the risk of decline in memory, possibly because of omega-3s in blood circulation. Curcumin, which is found in turmeric, has been shown to reduce amyloid plaques in the brain, therefore enabling better function.

Other treatments

Improvement of oral care. It is essential to take care of your teeth, gums and mouth, as swelling and infection in the gum can cause inflammatory responses through the body. To that end, regular dental check-ups and the use of an electric toothbrush and dental floss is recommended. Numerous studies have found a connection between poor oral hygiene and dementia. There is also an association between tooth loss and dementia. The risk increases by 1.4% with each additional tooth loss, though the use of dentures is also associated with dementia risk. However, those with dentures appeared to be at lower risk relative to individuals with uncorrected tooth loss. Bacteria associated with gum disease, such as p.gingivalis have been found in the brains of patients with Alzheimer's disease.

Step 2: There is a tendency for various hormones to decline with aging. Hormonal imbalance can influence the functioning of organs, including the brain. The hormonal levels most commonly affected are thyroid and oestrogen. Hormone replacement therapy can be used to balance out the levels of each hormone and optimise their performance in the body but may not be necessary to restore memory.

Treatment: Test hormone levels. Full hormone assessment should be carried out to determine if there are any imbalances that may be present. These include: thyroid profile, steroids such as cortisol, oestrogen, and testosterone. If hormonal imbalance is detected on the investigations, then the imbalance should be treated.

Treatment: Stress reduction

Methods to help one relax and destress are important. Stress is known to have a major impact on your body. Uncontrolled stress can lead to several dangerous medical conditions, including heart disease and even decline in memory. Daily meditation, yoga and using music to relax are all recommended treatments for stress.

Supplemental treatment

Supplements such as vitamin D3 and ashwagandha are recommended. It is now known that those with a deficiency of vitamin D are twice as likely to develop Alzheimer's disease. Ashwagandha is known to prevent beta- amyloid plaques from forming in the brain, thereby reducing symptoms of Alzheimer's.

Step 3: Optimise antioxidants

Research shows that when fats are oxidised in the brain there is a strong relationship with the development of Alzheimer's disease. Thus, optimisation of antioxidants will reduce and possibly prevent this from occurring and would therefore be protective against Alzheimer's disease. Antioxidants such as vitamin C and beta-carotene can therefore be preventative. In this regard, fresh citrus fruits, cherries and other sources rich in vitamin C can be protective. One should be wary of using tap water for drinking purposes because of its chlorine content. The water suppliers defence for adding chlorine to our water supplies is to help to keep the water free from disease causing organisms. This very chlorine, though, because of its potent oxidising ability, is able to lead to oxidation of fats in the brain which increases our risk of Alzheimer's disease.

Treatment: Diet

A cup of blueberries each day is a useful addition to one's diet. Spinach, kale, oranges and other foods high in beta-carotene or vitamin C should be able to reduce the rate of memory decline.

Supplemental treatments

Supplemental treatments here are vitamin E, selenium, vitamin C, N-acetylcysteine and alpha-lipoic acid. Research tells us that individuals with a low level of vitamin E are more prone to develop Alzheimer's. Selenium helps to protect the nerve cell function in the brain, thereby preventing memory loss. N-acetylcysteine protects the nerve cells by acting as an anti-inflammatory agent in the brain. Alpha-lipoic acid is a powerful antioxidant that can effectively slow down the progress of Alzheimer's disease.

Step 4: Optimise gut health

Healthy gut flora is essential for brain function. Gut health is essential for managing many different medical illnesses.

Treatment: Diets based on whole, healthy foods eliminating grains, carbohydrates and sugars help to prevent upset of gut flora and so optimise gut health.

Treatment supplements: Probiotics can be used to supplement gut health. Probiotics break down to gamma-aminobutyric acid (GABA). GABA is a neurotransmitter in the brain and its deficiency leads to a decline in memory and dementia.

Step 5: Plenty of healthy fats

General advice is that we should stay away from harmful fats, but there are some essential fats for your health. Healthy fats are needed to maintain healthy brain function. Unhealthy fats include fats found in dairy, eggs and meat. Healthy fats are those that are polyunsaturated and monounsaturated, and include fats obtained from avocado, olives, seeds and nuts. Healthy fats play an integral role in the production of acetylcholine, a major neurotransmitter which is essential for learning, concentration and memory.

Treatment: Apart from DHA and EPA mentioned above, another recommended fat is found in coconut oils called medium chain triglycerides (MCT oils)

Step 6: Enhancing cognitive performance and NGF (nerve growth factor) levels

Recommended supplements include lion's mane (Hericium erinaceus), mushroom extract, Bacopa monnieri and citicoline. Lion's mane is a mushroom which has been shown to have positive effects on how the brain works. Bacopa is a herb used in Indian medicine to treat memory problems; when tried on humans, there were improvements in maintaining attention and verbal recall. Citicoline is a substance present in the brain which increases the production of phosphatidylcholine which plays an important role in brain function.

Step 7: Boost mitochondrial function

A contributing factor to Alzheimer's disease is the slowing down of brain cells' activity. This can be attributed to the powerhouse of the cells called mitochondria. With mitochondrial dysfunction the ability of the brain to work effectively in areas of memory declines. This should be easily treatable with supplements.

Treatment: Supplements

The supplements recommended for this are pyrroloquinoline quinone (PQQ) and coenzyme Q10 (CoQ10). In Alzheimer's there is often an accumulation of a protein called amyloid in the brain and PQQ tends to reduce the amount of amyloid formed. CoQ10 is associated with memory improvements.

Step 8: Mental and physical exercise

Mental and physical exercise are essential requirements such as crossword puzzles, Sudoku or any type of activity that requires memory.

Mental and physical exercise is an essential requirement in maintaining our health. Physical exercise is vital to keep blood circulating throughout our bodies to carry oxygen and nourishment to cells and tissues whilst removing the waste produced by these very organs and tissues.

Treatment: Mental exercise

Any type of mental exercise is helpful. Suggestions of crossword puzzles, Sudoku, or any type of activity that requires memory and recall. It has been shown that simply exercising your brain keeps brain cells alive and by extension helps to keep Alzheimer's disease and dementia at bay.

Treatment: Physical exercise

We suggest a minimum of 30 minutes – better to do 60 minutes of physical exercise daily. Strength training or low-impact cardio exercise should be undertaken between 4 and 6 times each week. Low-impact and strength training is less strenuous on the body but will increase blood flow to the brain and other vital organs.

Step 9: Ensure nocturnal oxygenation

Nocturnal oxygenation refers to the amount of oxygen your brain receives during the night while you are asleep. Sleep not only refers to the time spent with your eyes closed, but also includes the quality of sleep. There are some medical problems which interfere with breathing while you are sleeping and thus starve your brain of oxygen.

Treatment: Sleep

The brain needs oxygen to function properly, so any shortage on the supply of oxygen to the brain will impact on brain function. One reasonably common condition called apnea can interfere with the supply of oxygen to the brain. This can be reasonably well treated with the use of a CPAP machine. This requires you to use a face mask while you sleep and forces air into your lungs. Excessive snoring can be a sign that you may be suffering from sleep apnea.

Step 10: Detoxification of heavy metals

Metals considered as heavy metals include lead, arsenic, cadmium, mercury, aluminium, uranium, strontium and thallium. Some of these compounds may sound foreign to you, but I will include some of the more common entities on this list. Lead is commonly found in our drinking water supplies, having found its way there through our lead pipes, faucets and plumbing fixtures. Arsenic is a common ingredient in rat poison and can enter the body in food and water; it may also enter the body when we swallow soil or dust. Cadmium enters the body from smoking tobacco, eating, and drinking food and water containing cadmium, and inhaling it from the air. Mercury can enter our body from eating fish containing methylmercury or exposure to high levels of elemental mercury vapour. Dental amalgams are also known to be a source of mercury to the human being, albeit in low doses and mainly at the times of installation and removal. Aluminium enters our bodies through our respiratory tract; a small amount enters through the food and water we consume, and a small amount from antacids. These heavy metals are ubiquitous and enter our bodies through a variety of portals. Research tells us that getting rid of these heavy metals from the blood will prevent Alzheimer's symptoms from becoming worse or even developing.

Treatment: Detox

Chelation therapy is the only known method currently available for the removal of heavy metals from the blood and, by extension, the body. We would encourage that the use of chelation therapy be done under medical supervision.

Pause For Thought

- What is the ICT?
- Does the ICT work?
- What is involved in the ICT?
- Does eating less than 3 hours before bedtime have any implications for Alzheimer's disease?
- Could fasting for 12 hours between dinner and breakfast be helpful?
- What is the value of sleep in maintaining brain health?
- Can weight loss be useful in the prevention and management of Alzheimer's disease?
- Can nutritional supplements be helpful in treating the Alzheimer's patient?

Take Home Nuggets

- A workable approach in treating and preventing the progressive development of Alzheimer's disease is the ICT protocol, this involves a preliminary full evaluation of the patient, involving a series of blood studies. This is not based on a one size fits all approach, It is individualised.

- This approach has been shown to be effective in many studies and has led to individuals recovering sufficiently to return to full time employment and even pursuing other learning activities.

- This is a ten-step protocol which recommends among other things

- avoidance of food for at least three hours before bed and a 12 hour fast between dinner and breakfast.

- It also recommends the use of dietary supplements. Obtaining your

- ideal body weight is also useful.

- The value of 7-8 hours of sleep is not overrated because of the cleansing of the brain which takes place at this time.

Notes

_____

_____

_____

_____

_____

_____

_____

_____

_____

_____

_____

_____

_____

_____

_____

_____

_____

_____

_____

_____

_____

Notes

_____

_____

_____

_____

_____

_____

_____

_____

_____

_____

_____

_____

_____

_____

_____

_____

_____

_____

_____

Chapter 5
Alzheimer's Disease: Do We Know the Root Cause? What Does the Science Tell Us?

- Determining the cause

- Environmental toxins and our vulnerable brain

- Which are the culpable heavy metals?

- Brain's natural protective mechanism

- Enhancing methylation

- Pause For Thought

- Take Home Nuggets

- Pages for personal notes

Alzheimer's disease, as indicated above, was diagnosed at post-mortem after the brain of an individual who presented with then unfamiliar memory diminution and unusual behaviour was examined. We were now aware of the changes in the brain of individuals displaying similar characteristics, and the science has now evolved to a place where imaging studies can help in the diagnosis of this condition. The determination of the causative factors, as in much of science, however, still lags behind.

Most would, however, posit that knowledge of the cause of a disease is 50% of the process in finding a cure; so, it is with this belief that understanding the root cause of this disease is integral to understanding proposed cures.

We are aware of the familial relationship among Alzheimer's sufferers, so it is not uncommon that the usual forgetfulness seen among aged pensioners is linked with this awful disease. It is clearly obvious that the litany of drugs used in conventional medicine have not been very effective. About twelve years ago I was informed that one of my ex-girlfriends had been diagnosed with Alzheimer's; initially, I did not believe it and asked the person communicating this information to desist from these comments. Unfortunately, she was correct, and I was able to observe first-hand some of the debilitating effects of this disease. This has driven my curiosity into researching this disease process to not only protect myself, but also explore preventative measures which have been shown to allay this condition. I will share some of my findings with you, hoping that you, too, can be given usable nuggets that will protect you from this devastating condition.

As shocking as it may seem, the root cause of this condition may be already known and is entirely supported by medical literature.

Among the drugs used to treat Alzheimer's disease, only Aricept and Namenda, at best, can slow down the progress of the disease. The other treatments offered are analogous to Band-Aids that have to be used for ever. The simple explanation is that they do not address the root cause of memory loss and Alzheimer's.

Environmental toxins and our vulnerable brain

Environmental toxins are the leading cause of neurological illness. Although our bodies are built to protect our brains from these toxic assaults, intermittently these built-in protection systems may be defective and hence fail to provide effective elimination of these toxins. Depending on the extent of this defect, one can understand why one toxin will have a specific effect on one person but have little or no effect on another person. Unfortunately for us our bodies are continuously exposed to toxins which have an additive effect at the cellular level. Current Alzheimer's research reveals that these environmental toxins alter metabolic pathways associated with the development and progression of the disease, thereby confirming the root cause of this disease. This points an indisputable finger at the heavy metal industries which encourage a wave of Alzheimer's and other neurological diseases.

What are the culpable heavy metals?

In the previous chapter we listed a few heavy metals which are known to be toxic to the neurological system, and here we name three common heavy metals. These are mercury, aluminium and copper. We indicated how these heavy metals gain access to our bodies and create their havoc on our neurological systems and memory loss. Let us revisit mercury. Mercury is believed to be one of the major contributors to the impact of heavy metals on the brain. High levels of mercury in the brain lead to two brain abnormalities associated with Alzheimer's disease: neurofibrillary tangles and amyloid plaques. Interestingly, the mercury levels in the brains of Alzheimer's patients are at least three times the rest of the population. Although the source of this mercury is mainly fish and other seafoods, those are not the only source, and though I am not advocating this, even if we eliminate fish from our diet, we will still be exposed to mercury. This is mainly because the coal-burning industry is pumping out a staggering 48 tons of mercury into the air every year.

Aluminium has been known to have a deleterious effect on the brain for more than 20 years. We ingest 7–9mg of aluminium daily. Apart from the amount we ingest daily, we continue to expose ourselves to aluminium through our continued use of antiperspirants, cooking with aluminium utensils and ingesting aluminium containing drugs and vaccines.

Though not mentioned in the previous chapter, copper is another such heavy metal which presents a growing threat as the amount of this heavy metal in our environment is skyrocketing. The increased exposure to this heavy metal is particularly disturbing since it has been shown to be toxic to the neurological system and has been specifically linked to Alzheimer's disease. That is not all, as high copper levels have been found to destroy essential detoxifying nutrients including vitamins C and B, and zinc. A word of caution to ladies using birth control, such as the copper-T coil: these preparations can raise the copper levels in your body.

If a blood test for these metals reveals that you have high levels, then a detoxification plan can be devised by your medical team.

Brain's natural protective mechanism

The brain has a protective mechanism which seeks to protect us from the toxic effects of such heavy metals. Coming to the fore is the amino acid glutathione. This amino acid is often referred to as the master antioxidant and is a powerful detoxifier and immune system enhancer that serves as the main antioxidant protectant of the entire body.

Glutathione is both produced and regenerated through a process called methylation that is responsible for immune system function, neurotransmitter production, organ protection and detoxification.

During the methylation process, genetically controlled enzymes, specifically methylenetetrahydrofolate reductase (MTHFR), are critical to the methylation process. It uses vitamin B and other nutrients to produce an endless supply of glutathione when things work well. So, with individuals who are unable to produce adequate quantities of glutathione, it may be because of genetic defects, and they will be unable to adequately protect themselves against the toxic effects of these heavy metals, leading to memory loss and possibly Alzheimer's disease and dementia. Armed with this information we can treat these patients with nutrients which aim to enhance methylation.

Enhancing methylation

CerefolinNAC is a powerful brain supplement which is aimed at helping to prevent Alzheimer's and memory loss. This preparation was developed to target the toxic damage that is linked to memory loss. CerefolinNAC contains vitamin

B12 and folic acid, as well as the potent amino acid N-acetylcysteine (NAC), a known glutathione producer. This is believed to aid the liver in genetically bypassing methylation defects so that your body can produce quantitative amounts of glutathione. This preparation is doubtlessly pricey, so an alternative can be the combination of vitamin B, NAC, alpha-lipoic acid, zinc and selenium.

Pause For Thought

- What is the cause of Alzheimer's disease?
- Is the cause known?
- Can metabolic toxins contribute to the cause of Alzheimer's disease?
- Which heavy metals are associated with Alzheimer's disease?
- What is the role of glutathione in brain protection?
- Can the combination of vitamin B, N-acetyl cysteine, alpha lipoic acid, zinc and selenium help?

Take Home Nuggets

- All the causes of Alzheimer's disease are not known, but there are some which are known and in treatment of the condition we need to address the known causes.
- Environmental toxins are involved and are believed to alter metabolic pathways and the subsequent result is the development of Alzheimer's disease.

- Heavy metals such as mercury, aluminium and copper are also suspects in the cause of this disease.

- Glutathione is an amino acid which plays an important role in protecting the brain.

- A combination of Vitamin B, N- acetylcysteine, alpha lipoic acid, zinc and selenium is effective therapy against the ravages of Alzheimer's disease.

Notes

_____

_____

_____

_____

_____

_____

_____

_____

_____

_____

_____

_____

_____

_____

_____

_____

_____

_____

_____

Notes

_____

_____

_____

_____

_____

_____

_____

_____

_____

_____

_____

_____

_____

_____

_____

_____

_____

_____

_____

_____

_____

Chapter 6
Minerals to the Rescue

- What of lithium?
- Further benefits of lithium usage
- The value of sleep
- What do animal studies tell us?
- Pause For Thought
- Take Home Nuggets
- Pages for personal notes

Much of the clinical experience with lithium, a known mineral, has been in the treatment of patients who experience bipolar disorder. The unasked question until recently was just how is lithium able to produce this effect? We have failed to take advantage of the brain-protective and brain anti- aging effects of low-dose lithium.

A ground-breaking study published in the Proceedings of the National Academy of Sciences shows that it can halt the progression of degenerative neurone disease.

Lithium is best described as a mineral element in the same group of the periodic table as sodium and potassium. It is not classified as a drug and so not patentable but has enormous potential for protecting and improving brain health. Using MRI scans researchers have been able to show that lithium increases the number of brain cells in older individuals, and so lithium has been credited with increasing human brain grey matter, and has also been found to stimulate progenitor proliferation which promotes the growth of new nerve cells.

Lithium seems capable of launching a three-pronged protective envelope against the most common brain-destroyers. It has been shown to have a neuroprotective effect against focal shortage of oxygen in rats. It has also been shown to exhibit robust neuroprotective effects in the central nervous system. This protective effect not only is restricted to external toxins including aluminium, but also relates to internally produced molecules which are toxic to nerve cells such as glutamate. Researchers have also been able to show that lithium protects brain cells not only against toxins, but also against lack of blood flow.

At least one way in which lithium is able to offer neuroprotection is by increasing levels of a major neuroprotective protein called "Bcl-2". This compound Bcl-2 also increases regeneration of parts of the nerve cell called axons. Axons are projections from the main body of nerve cells that contact other neurons.

Further benefits to lithium usage

Lithium inhibits amyloid secretion in cells transfected with amyloid precursor proteins. It also protects neurons against beta-amyloid-induced neurodegeneration. It must be remembered that both amyloid and beta- amyloid are by-products of nerve cell metabolism that, in excess, contribute to Alzheimer's disease. Others have been able to demonstrate that lithium prevents the formation of neurofibrillary tangles, a pathognomonic finding in the brains of those suffering from Alzheimer's disease. A study from the Indiana University School of Medicine has vouched for lithium as a treatment for Alzheimer's disease.

I recommend a dose of 5-10mg daily (do not exceed 20mg) of lithium as an aspartate or orotate daily. Warning: lithium can be dangerous in high doses, so please be guided on the suggested dosage described on the package.

Lithium has been found to be effective in treating other behaviour and diseases which have a neural component. For example, it has been successfully used to treat mood disturbances, addiction, and alcoholism. Recently it has been shown to effectively slow down the progression of amyotrophic lateral sclerosis, also referred to as ALS or Lou Gehrig's disease. The moniker Lou Gehrig's disease was derived from the home- run-hitting major league American baseball player Lou Gehrig after he was diagnosed with the condition in 1939. Gehrig deteriorated very rapidly after his diagnosis. In fact, less than two years after his initial symptoms of weakness and stumbling appeared, he died totally paralysed and helpless. ALS is a devastating neurodegenerative disorder with no effective treatment. Daily doses of lithium delayed disease progression in human patients affected by ALS. It is noteworthy that in comparing lithium to one of the more common treatments for ALS, riluzole, it was observed that the patients treated with riluzole experienced an average symptom worsening of 50% in just three months, and 30% of the patients treated with riluzole died within 15 months. In contrast, none of the patients treated with lithium died in the fifteen months of the study, and none of them experienced a deterioration in their condition.

Before embarking on self-treatment, we advise that you discuss your source and plans with your doctor.

The value of sleep

I need not continue to extol the virtues of a good night's sleep, but just what does sleep have to do with brain disease? Our day-to-day experience helps us to realise that we are less productive if we do not get an adequate night's rest. We may be able to function, but our productivity declines. With no sleep in a 24-hour period we spend the following day in an almost drunken stupor. We also realise that the more elderly around us tend to get by on less sleep per night. We watch as they stumble through the day and attribute their stumbles to growing older, trying to reassure anyone who would listen that these are among the signs associated with getting older. We observe their continuous decline in their memory and their powers of recall, again attributing this to be normally associated with aging. Currently, we know from research that good sleep is critical for the proper functioning of our immune system. We have learned that a major component of our immune system, the T cells, plummet when we are sleep-deprived: this is true irrespective of our health status.

In addition to its effects on lymphocytes and other white blood cells, sleep deprivation raises the level of inflammatory messengers in one's body. People who are sleep-deprived have higher levels of interleukin-6 and inflammatory markers such as C-reactive protein (CRP). If unchecked, this inflammation will have serious health consequences and contribute to heart disease, cancer, and brain disease like Alzheimer's. I am not for a minute suggesting that lack of sleep causes Alzheimer's disease, but could there be more to a good night sleep, than simply protection against Alzheimer's disease and adding years to one's life?

What do animal studies tell us?

Dr Maiken Nedergaard, the sleep biologist who runs the Sleep Centre at the University of Rochester, has, with her team, studied the role of sleep in one's body. They concluded that sleep is the body's way of cleansing your brain. Our bodies have a cleansing system called a lymphatic system which travels through our bodies through lymph channels carrying macrophages and other immune cells that can engulf debris and the toxic products of metabolism.

Unfortunately, these cleansing lymph cells are unable to cross the blood-brain barrier to reach the brain. The blood-brain barrier describes a network of blood vessels and tissue that is made up of closely spaced cells, and functions in keeping harmful substances from reaching the brain. The blood-brain barrier lets some substances, such as water, oxygen, carbon dioxide and general anaesthetics, pass into the brain.

The brain uses one-fifth of the total energy used by the body to perform its critical role. With that amount of energy expenditure, a lot of waste is inevitably created. Some of this waste, like tau proteins and beta-amyloid plaques, are toxic to the brain and will lead to Alzheimer's and other types of dementia if they are not removed.

While we are awake, our brains are too active to be involved in self- cleaning. There is, however, a cleaning mechanism involving glial cells which functions in moving through the fluid spaces in our brains during the day. These glial cells only clean the surface of the brain while we are awake. In Dr Nedergaard's work she used tagged markers which were injected into the cerebrospinal fluid of mice, and these tagged markers were tracked. These markers were found to follow specific pathways through the brain and out again. When the mice were asleep, however, the fluid exchange increased 20-fold.

How is that possible? It appears that while we are asleep our brain's organic matter shrinks (a physiological shrinkage); this leads to an expansion of the channels between the cells, allowing more cerebrospinal to circulate around individual cells carrying more glial cells, and thus providing a medium for the cleansing glial cells to move in and around each cell, removing any debris that they come across. The researchers measured a 60% increase in the flow through interstitial fluid over that seen when the mice were awake. It is therefore obvious that the sleeping brain clears twice as much waste as the same brain when awake. Much of this waste was identified as beta-amyloid, the toxic substance linked to the development of Alzheimer's disease, thus arguing for the beneficial effects of sleep since this is the time when the brain cleans itself.

Pause For Thought

- Is there any value to the use of lithium in the treatment of Alzheimer's disease?

- Does lithium increase the number of brain cells?

- Can lithium protect the brain from oxygen shortages?

- Can any mineral limit amyloid secretion?

- What is amyloid? What happens when it is produced in excessive quantities?

- Can getting 7-8 hours of sleep per night aid brain health?

- Why does the volume of cerebrospinal fluid circulating in the brain increase 20-fold while we are asleep?

Take Home Nuggets

- Lithium has long been known as a treatment for patients who suffer from bipolar affective disorder, more recently lithium has been shown to increase the number of brain cells. It is also able to protect brain cells from oxygen shortages. It has also been shown that lithium limits amyloid secretion in the brain and therefore can protect against Alzheimer's development and manifestations.

- Although during sleep brain activity is not as pronounced as during our periods of wakefulness, it has been shown that the circulation in the brain of cerebrospinal fluid increases 20-fold during sleep. Why you may ask? We believe that this is the time when the brain cleanses itself of toxins and other debris which can impact on its health. Hence sleeping for 7 to 8 hours per night can delay and possibly prevent the development of Alzheimer's disease as well as other types of dementia.

Notes

_____

_____

_____

_____

_____

_____

_____

_____

_____

_____

_____

_____

_____

_____

_____

_____

_____

_____

_____

_____

_____

_____

_____

_____

Notes

Chapter 7
Lessons from Nature

- Plausible link between Alzheimer's disease and an infectious aetiology

- Evidence for this link between Alzheimer's disease and Herpes simplex virus-1?

- Could moulds be culpable?

- Has nature provided us with therapy?

- Pause For Thought

- Take Home Nuggets

- Pages for personal notes

There are some who believe that with every disease, there is a naturally occurring cure. Does this apply to brain disease? Let's explore the role of mould, the human herpes simplex virus and a specific mushroom, and test this hypothesis.

Recently a psychiatrist from Colorado by the name of Theodore Henderson, an MD/PhD, wrote an article in which he linked Alzheimer's disease with a relatively common virus, herpes simplex virus-1 (HSV-1). It is alleged that having a single cold sore at any time in your life increases your chance of having Alzheimer's disease. This is very important news as Alzheimer's disease is on the increase. Currently there are over 5 million in the USA with a diagnosis of

Alzheimer's disease. This number does not include the cohort who are classified as having mild cognitive impairment, considered by some to be a pre-Alzheimer's state. The outlook is grim when one recognises that current treatment options offered by traditional medicine have little or no impact on the disease process.

The claim that there is a link between Alzheimer's disease and herpes simplex virus is not far-fetched when one realises that some viruses are known to hide and live in the nervous system.

The chickenpox virus, for example, lives in the nerves of the nervous system and it reappears along the root of the nerve that stems from the spinal cord in which it was hiding. Some genital herpes sufferers will experience a tingling around the tailbone or back which mirrors the site in which the virus is hiding most of the time.

For the purpose of clarification, we have two types of herpes simplex virus (HSV), referred to as HSV-1, which tend to have their effect in the area of the face and head which is a short distance from the brain, and HSV-2, which has its effect in the genital area. It seems feasible that the HSV-1 virus can make the short journey to the brain when activated. Since this virus tends to become active during episodes of immune compromise, if someone's immune system is suppressed, the virus can slowly cause permanent damage to the brain, leading to Alzheimer's disease.

Evidence for this link between Alzheimer's disease and Herpes simplex virus-1?

There are several scientific studies which make a strong connection between HSV-1 and Alzheimer's disease.

In summary:

- Multiple studies show a positive correlation between HSV-1 showing up in blood work and the incidence of Alzheimer's.

- At least three studies show that autopsies have found the DNA of HSV-1 in the tangles and plaques in the brains of both humans and animals with Alzheimer's.

- HSV-1 is more prominently found in the places of the brain that are damaged (the frontal and temporal lobes).

- Three studies show HSV-1 induces the formation of the classic plaques seen in Alzheimer's patients when injected into tissue in a laboratory Petri dish.

- A study in 2011 showed that when antiviral medication was placed in test tubes with nerve cells that had the classic plaque and sticky proteins of the disease, the disease process was slowed down, and stopped the production of, and even erased the classic signs of, Alzheimer's disease in those tissues.

This is frightening since about 34% of the population has antibodies to this virus, but some sources say that the figure is closer to 90%, since one may have been exposed to HSV-1, have it in their system but not know it.

On first exposure to the virus, be it through sharing a drinking utensil or even kissing your lady friend, your immune system may have been sufficiently robust to have the virus sequestered. So, although you may be free of symptoms, you may be a carrier of the virus.

With this volume of information revealing the correlation between HSV-1 and Alzheimer's disease, is it time to request that an antiviral agent such as acyclovir be added to the brew in trying to treat patients affected by this dreaded disease? Alternatively, can we screen these patients for HSV-1 antibodies: if present can we take a two-pronged targeted approach by which we slow down the activity of the virus with supplements such as garlic, grapefruit seed extract, oil of oregano and olive leaf extract, or even the amino acid lysine (at a dose of 1,000–3,000mg a day). The second prong of this fight is to strengthen our immune system. Those who suffer from cold sores will generally observe specific trigger factors such as physical and mental stress, poor sleep, and poor diet and maybe too much sugar. A suggested approach to keeping your immune system strong would be the use of 20mg of zinc and 1000mg of vitamin C daily over a prolonged period. This may prove magical in strengthening your immune system and allow you to fight off a range of infections.

Could moulds be culpable?

From time to time, I am sure that you have questioned whether your home makes you ill. You feel lethargic, unusually fatigued, unable to think clearly, and are almost always having to cope with health challenges, flu, allergies, hay fever, the common cold etc. You leave this home and get out on a holiday, even if locally, and almost instantly you start feeling refreshed. So, could your home be causing your health issues? It may, and mould may be the culprit.

In the UK, mould is a sufficient health threat that the advisory is once the problem of mould has been reported, the landlord has to respond within 14 days. Landlords are required to arrange a property inspection to determine the cause of the mould and, where necessary, repairs need to be made.

Awaab's Law will force social landlords to fix damp and mould within strict time limits, in a new amendment to the Social Housing (Regulation) Bill. There are new powers allowing the Housing Ombudsman to help landlords improve performance, in the amendments to the Social Housing (Regulation) Bill.

Mould is comprised of living organisms, and these are classified as fungi, which like other living organisms are driven to grow and expand. These living organisms produce toxins with a twofold intention: (a) to protect themselves, and (b) to challenge and weaken their immediate environment, thus making it easier for them to spread. It would seem with that ability, moulds are provided with a powerful tool that ensures their survival, but simultaneously is toxic to their immediate environment. Mould can be present and wreak havoc on the health of individuals even when it may not be readily visible. It is not uncommon to encounter mould growing in the walls of a building because of incorrect plumbing etc., but although not immediately visible to the naked eye, the toxins they produce will negatively impact on the health of the individual within the vicinity of the mould growth.

Mould is virtually ubiquitous and is considered by some to be a hidden killer as it is responsible for about 13 million infections and 1.5 million deaths globally annually as it grows in walls, attics and basements. It is estimated that some 40% of all American households are contaminated with some form of fungus.

Mould toxins irritate the brain and central nervous system causing a myriad of seemingly unrelated symptoms, including but not limited to:

- Fatigue
- Headaches
- Twitching
- Tremors
- Brain fog
- Muscle spasms and pain
- Insomnia
- Abdominal pains
- Frequent respiratory tract infections such as common colds.

Though exposure to mould is not good for anyone, some people are allergic to it, and in others it can cause severe symptoms if they have specific genetic susceptibility. Continuous exposure to mould at home, work or school can cause severe neurological diseases. It must be understood that all moulds are toxic to human beings, whether they are green, brown, or black. Some people can excrete the mould toxins if they are inhaled with insignificant consequences. There are others, however, who may be genetically handicapped and can't rid their bodies of the mould toxins. These toxins continue to build up, leading to health-eroding symptoms.

This insidious health hazard may present itself unannounced but create immeasurable havoc on our health that may be difficult to diagnose. In fact, only a few people receive the correct diagnosis even after destruction of their health by this fungus. A diagnosis can be readily made by having your doctor run a human leukocyte antigen (HLA) genetic test which looks specifically at the HLA or immune response gene.

Alternatively, there is a visual contrast sensitivity (VCS) test, also known as functional acuity contrast test (FACT), to evaluate how well your eye distinguishes contrast, black versus white, and your night vision. Information on mould toxicity can be found on the website www. survivingMould.com.

Other labs such as Realtime Laboratories (website: www.realtimelab. com) and BioTrek Laboratories (website: biotreklabs.com) specialise in urinary testing for mould toxins.

Has nature provided us with therapy?

There are thousands of varieties of mushroom growing in different areas of the world which are known to have a variety of medicinal benefits. There is this unusual-looking mushroom which has impressive medicinal benefits. It has shown tremendous benefits to those battling mood disorders, dementia and even Alzheimer's. It is believed to be capable of protecting the brain, allowing one to keep his/her memories intact throughout his life.

This mushroom is commonly called lion's mane. This mushroom does not look like the typical mushroom, and it has no cap; instead, it has long shafts called spines which hang down and have earned it names such as the bearded tooth and pom-pom mushroom. It is felt by some that this mushroom by DLiPE a staple in the treatment of a range of neurological illnesses, not least dementia and Alzheimer's. Traditional Chinese medicine has used the lion's mane for its antioxidant effects in treating stomach ailments and cancer. Recent discovery has improved our understanding of its impact on the brain. Its effect on the brain is believed to be caused by the presence of a group of compounds called hericenones. At least 8 of these hericenones have been discovered and found to have remarkable potential for the neurological system.

Hericenones can stimulate the production of nerve growth factor (NGF): this is a protein produced in the body which is critical for communication between nerve cells and the brain.

NGF is necessary for brain cells to function and to heal, and it has an important role in the activity and survival of spinal cord sensory neurons and the cholinergic neurons of the brain stem.

Studies in which mice were deprived of NGF led to an increase in the production of beta-amyloids and cell death, as well as the development of Alzheimer's-like dementia.

Thoughts of administering NGF by mouth or through the veins have been shelved because NGF cannot cross the blood-brain barrier, so it would be unable to reach the brain where it is most needed to bring about the desired effect for

Alzheimer's sufferers. The compounds found in lion's mane are sufficiently small to cross the blood-brain barrier where they can bring about the desired effects within the brain.

Hericenones also reduce the cell damage caused by amyloid peptides which have a known association with Alzheimer's disease. Hericenones seem to lessen the death of neurons and other brain cells. A human study in 2009 gave interesting results. 30 men and women aged between 50 and 80 years with mild cognitive impairment were studied in a double-blinded, placebo-controlled trial. Half the group were given powdered lion's mane, and the other half placebo. When tested at 12 and 16 weeks, the cognitive function of the treated group improved significantly, compared to the placebo group. When the therapy with lion's mane was stopped after 16 weeks, the benefits disappeared within a month.

A fat-soluble phospholipid molecule extracted from lion's mane' is called dilinoleoyl-phosphatidylethanolamine or DLiPE for short. Remove can be extracted from lion's mane. DLiPE appears to protect brain cells from oxidative damage that could lead to cell death in many neurodegenerative diseases such as Alzheimer's, Parkinson's and even bovine spongiform encephalopathy (mad cow disease). It would appear that these compounds present in Lion's mane' may be capable of reversing the effects of Alzheimer's disease.

There is also research evidence indicating that lion's mane powder offers benefits to people with mood disturbances, schizophrenia and depression. This product is available on Amazon, but can also be sourced from Mushroom Matrix, website: www.mushroommatrix.com.

Pause For Thought

- Is there a relationship between herpes simplex 1 and Alzheimer's disease?
- Can viruses live in neurons without showing any symptoms of disease for periods of time?
- How many types of Herpes simplex viruses are known to affect mankind?
- Can mould cause health issues?
- What is Awaab's law?
- What are the two motives of toxins produced by moulds?
- What is Lion Mane'?
- What are Hericenones?
- Is there any evidence that a special mushroom can be helpful in treating Alzheimer's patients?

Take Home Nuggets

It has been shown recently that even one infection with herpes simplex type 1 may be associated with the development of Alzheimer's disease. There are several studies which link HSV-1 to the development of Alzheimer's disease. It is believed that about 34% of the population has been exposed to HSV type 1, although some put the figure at 90%. This is the virus which causes cold sore whereas HSV type 2 affects the genital area.

Moulds are classified as fungi; they produce toxins with the dual aim of helping them to survive and weakening other organisms in their immediate environment so they can spread. Moulds causes inflammation of the central nervous system causing individuals to feel unwell.

Lion's Mane, a mushroom which has been shown to be useful in the treatment of several brain disorders. It contains a substance called hericenones. About eight different hericenones have been isolated which among other things increases the production of nerve growth factor (NGF) in our bodies. NGF is necessary for brain cells to function and to heal, and it has an important role in the activity and survival of spinal cord sensory neurons and the cholinergic neurons of the brain stem.

Notes

_____

_____

_____

_____

_____

_____

_____

_____

_____

_____

_____

_____

_____

_____

_____

_____

_____

_____

_____

_____

_____

Notes

_____

_____

_____

_____

_____

_____

_____

_____

_____

_____

_____

_____

_____

_____

_____

_____

_____

_____

_____

_____

_____

_____

Chapter 8
HRT and Alzheimer's Disease/Dementia

- Association between dementia and age

- The typical menopausal patient

- Common symptoms of the menopause

- HRT: A closer look

- The value of oestrogen in a female's life

- The role of oestrogen in the prepubertal phase

- The role of oestrogen in phase 2 of a lady's life

- The value of the oestrogen component

- The role of testosterone

- Oestrogen and the effect on the brain

- Pause For Thought

- Take Home Nuggets

- Pages for personal notes

Dementia affects more women than men. The obvious question is why? One may try to argue that women generally have a longer life span than men. Yes, it is true that women generally have a longer life span than men. Women over the age of 80 years may be more likely to have Alzheimer's disease than men of the same age. Interesting as that may be, it is even more instructive to learn that there are about twice as many women over age 65 with Alzheimer's as there are men over age 65 years with this condition. Worryingly though, the World Health Organisation (WHO) estimates that after we turn 60 years of age, 5% to 8% of us will live with dementia at some point. This would mean that after age 60 women are twice as likely to develop dementia/Alzheimer's like symptoms than men. The quoted age by the WHO is instructive. Women in that age group are expected to be in the menopause. The average age of menopause in the United Kingdom is 51 years in the USA the average age of menopause is 51.4 years. The quoted age of 60 years by the WHO leaves one with no doubt that this age group of women are in the menopause and with 9 years after the average age of menopause, it includes even women who would have gone into the menopause late. It also argues that the residual effects of the premenopausal hormones would have been eliminated from the bodies of these women.

The average girl will get her first period around 12 years in the United Kingdom. In the United States of America (USA), the average age of a girl having her first period is 12.4 years. If a girl's starts her menstrual cycles (menarche) about age 12 and on average, she continues to have monthly menstrual cycles till age 51; the woman's body is bathed with the hormones of ovarian cycling for about 39 years. At the onset of menopause these hormones are withdrawn and are no more; so, after 39 years, the woman is simply forced to exist without the substances which were integral to her person for all of 39 years. We start seeing patients in our clinics with a variety of seemingly unrelated symptoms in the years leading up to the menopause and for several years after the menopause.

The typical menopausal patient

The typical menopausal patient presents with any or many of these complaints:

- My life is challenging, I am struggling to keep up with my daily activities

- My last period was in my forties.

- I cannot live like this; I am continuously sweating.

- When folks around me are feeling cold, I am burning up.

- I am always tired.

- Sleeping is near impossible.

- I think that I am unusually harsh to the husband and children, they claim that I always seem to be in a bad mood.

- I am unable to concentrate for any length of time, I find it very difficult completing a task and most of the time they are left incomplete. Learning new information is difficult and near impossible.

- I have no sex drive; my vagina is dry and feels like it is on fire.

- Moving is so painful, that I dread the thought of having to move, so exercise or even walking is virtually impossible.

Common Symptoms of the Menopause

Patients regularly complain of hot flushes, night sweats, vaginal dryness and discomfort during sex, difficulty sleeping, low mood and anxiety, mental fog, reduced sex drive (libido), problems with memory and concentration. Though these symptoms initially seem unrelated, with a supply of appropriate hormone replacement, these patients almost immediately experience relief of these seemingly unrelate symptoms. It is therefore not farfetched to believe that the hormones of the ovaries may be in some way protective of brain function, after all, low mood, anxiety, mental fog and problems with memory and focus are all associated with the menopause and is also seen in the Alzheimer's patient and are noticeably relieved with HRT.

HRT: A closer look

The ovary produces three basic hormones, oestrogen, progesterone, and testosterone. The bulk of HRT preparations on the market are composed of only oestrogen and progesterone, either in combination or oestrogen only. Rarely as in the case of tibolone is testosterone included as a component of the HRT preparation.

The general advice is that any female who still has her uterus must receive the combined HRT preparation, that is a preparation containing both oestrogen and progesterone. This is necessary since unopposed oestrogen has deleterious effects on the lining/endometrium of the uterus. In the endometrium, unopposed oestrogen induces proliferative or invasive changes which represent the initial stages of a variety of diseases. This includes an increased risk of endometrial hyperplasia, endometrial polyps, endometriosis, adenomyosis and endometrial cancer. The addition of progestogen reduces this risk but may cause unacceptable symptoms, such as bleeding and spotting. Not only does this affect compliance but it triggers other investigations which may be bothersome and stressful, because social dislocation in terms of trips to the hospital and the anxiety from the fear that they may have cancer. In patients with post-menopausal bleeding there is only a 10% risk of malignancy. Though in 90% of cases the findings may be benign, every patient presenting with post-menopausal bleeding needs to be investigated, the process doubtlessly increases anxiety and fear in these patients, dreading that they may have cancer. The encouraging element in all of this is endometrial cancer generally presents at a relatively early stage of the disease process with postmenopausal bleeding. The removal of the uterus by a hysterectomy generally leads to a cure, although these patients are kept under surveillance for several years to ensure there is no recurrence. The only reason for the addition of progesterone is to protect the endometrium in postmenopausal women requiring HRT.

The Value of Oestrogen in a female's life

Let us divide a woman's life into three phases: Phase (1): the prepubertal phase: the time from birth to her first menstrual period. Phase (2) the phase between the first menstrual period and menopause and phase (3) the phase from menopause to death. What role does oestrogen play in each of these phases? Let us explore.

The Role of Oestrogen in the prepubertal Phase

In girls, blood levels of oestradiol start to increase around eight years of age, in boys, testosterone levels increase typically at 9 years of age or later. The difference in blood sex hormones levels is evident in children above eight years. Prepubertal girls have approximately an eight-fold higher level of serum oestrogen than prepubertal boys. The pubertal growth spurt in both sexes is driven primarily by oestrogen. The more rapid maturation of the bones of prepubertal girls may be explained by their higher oestrogen levels.

In infancy the development is intriguing and is characterized an activation phase in the brain, the so called gonadotrope axis, for a short period just after birth. This is referred to as the 'mini puberty' by some. Many studies have shown that both sexes display high levels of follicle-stimulating hormone (FSH) and luteinizing hormone (LH) and a gender-specific elevation of sex steroid hormones (testosterone in males and oestradiol in females) after birth. There is higher FSH levels in girls than in boys and higher LH levels in boys than in girls. The postnatal elevation of testosterone levels in humans results in testicular descent in males, maturation of the testis, and penile growth. It may also influence the masculinisation of the brain, a process initiated during life in the womb and mediated by testosterone produced by developing testes. In male rodents, numerous studies, showed that the perinatal period (end of live in the womb and the first few days after birth) is critical for masculinisation and defeminisation of the nervous system. Ovarian activity is particularly elevated after birth, with an intense synthesis and release of hormones, such as oestrogens (oestrone (E1) and oestradiol (E2)). Their production depends upon the expression of steroidogenic enzymes, such as aromatase which ensures the conversion of androgens into oestrogens. This notable ovarian activity occurs in time with the development of structures related to reproductive success. Oestrogens may already act on several organs to influence their differentiation/maturation. The conservation of this phase among female mammals suggests that this transient gonadotrope axis activation is important for reproductive function. It would therefore seem that in the female, even while still in the womb oestrogen is the dominant female hormone.

The Role of oestrogen in Phase 2 of a lady's Life

Oestrogen is one of two sex hormones associated with females. Along with progesterone, oestrogen plays a key role in a woman's reproductive health. The development of the secondary sexual characteristics (breasts, hips, etc), menstruation, and pregnancy are all possible because of oestrogen. Oestrogen is therefore the major female sex hormone in her reproductive life.

Suddenly at the menopause, this is the hormone, oestrogen, to the withdrawal of which is most likely to have the greatest impact on the patient. Hormone replacement therapy must therefore include oestrogen. Oestrogen plays an important role in other body systems, too. Hence all genders make oestrogen. So why do we add progesterone?

The value of the oestrogen component

Patients are generally advised that once their uterus is retained, they will need a combined HRT preparation; a preparation which includes both oestrogen and progesterone. If the only logical explanation advanced for the use of a combined preparation is the retention of a patient's uterus, could this be a reason to suggest the removal of the uterus before the commencement of HRT in women requesting HRT.

The two common reasons advanced to limit the duration of the use of combined HRT is (a) the risk of breast cancer is increased and (b) there is an increased risk of venous thromboembolism. It now appears that this risk is true only for the combined preparation.

- Oestrogen-only HRT has several benefits to the menopausal women. Oestrogen replacement only reduces the severity and frequency of hot flushes by around 85%.

- Oestrogen improves vaginal dryness.

- Oestrogen improves sleep and quality of life.

- Oestrogen protects the bony skeleton thereby reducing the risk of post-menopausal bone fracture.

- Oestrogen also improves skin elasticity and induces the appearance of younger looking skin, making an individual look younger than their calendar age.

- Oestrogen also alleviates mental fog, anxiety, and low moods.

The Role of Testosterone

Ovaries do not only produce oestrogen and progesterone, but they produce a third hormone, testosterone. What is the role of testosterone in the postmenopausal female? Observational studies have shown correlations between higher testosterone levels and improved cardiovascular health, improve bone density and reduced the risk of hip fracture. During the menopause, women will experience decreased sex drive, increased fat mass and decreased lean mass. Replacing testosterone has been shown to improve mood and libido, increase muscle mass and decrease fat deposits.

One form of HRT mentioned above called tibolone has all the hormones generally produced by the ovaries, that is oestrogen, progesterone and testosterone which would be the ideal HRT since it mirrors the hormones produced by the ovaries. Unfortunately, tibolone has been banned because of the risk of endometrial, ovarian and breast cancer. It is believed that this risk is indirect and is due to the aromatisation or conversion of testosterone to oestrogen. The risk of breast cancer is no higher than for oestrogen only HRT users, and as mentioned above the oestrogen would trigger proliferative and invasive changes in the lining of the uterus.

Oestrogen and the effect on the Brain

Membrane-associated oestrogen receptors are found at several sites in the brain associated with learning and memory. Additionally, oestrogen plays an important regulatory function on different processes such as cognition, anxiety, body temperature, feeding and sexual behaviour. These findings argue for the effects of Oestrogen on the Alzheimer's patient.

Many preclinical studies have documented the manifold regulatory actions of ovarian steroids on neuronal biochemistry, cellular metabolism, and behaviour. Consistent with these findings were the ostensible beneficial effects of oestrogen on cognitive function and on the course of dementia, including Alzheimer's disease (AD), repeatedly reported in observational studies.

It is now being reported that one of the risks for Alzheimer's disease is oestrogen deficiency that may interfere with the extension of neurofibrillary tangles. There is mounting evidence that oestrogen may decrease hyperphosphorylated tau deposits in the brain.

Research has also shown that oestrogen may help to protect the brain from Alzheimer's by blocking some of the harmful effects of amyloid plaques which build up in Alzheimer's and causes brain cells to become damaged or die.

Interestingly, when both progesterone and oestrogen were given together, progesterone appears to hinder oestrogen 's main beneficial function: preventing the build up of beta amyloid protein, an important risk factor in the development of Alzheimer's disease.

A meta-analysis of seven studies with a total of 5251 older men, found that lower testosterone concentration in their bodies was associated with an increased risk of Alzheimer's disease.

The evidence is clear and strong that oestrogen replacement therapy and testosterone replacements in our aging population will help to reduce the onset of this most dreaded disease, Alzheimer's.

Pause For Thought

- Is Alzheimer's more common in women or men of the same age?
- What does the oestrogen receptors in our brain suggest?
- Can oestrogen only Hormone replacement protect against Alzheimer's disease?
- Does the combination of oestrogen and progesterone (combined HRT) protect against Alzheimer's disease?
- Can Testosterone replacement protect against Alzheimer's disease?
- Is a woman's body generally flushed with her ovarian hormones through-out her life?
- What is the average age of menopause in the UK?
- What is the average age of menopause in the USA?

Take Home Nuggets

- Alzheimer's disease is more common among women than men of identical age groups. It was thought that this was due to the longer life span of women, but it is now emerging that the ovarian hormones are protective against Alzheimer's disease. Testosterone is also protective against Alzheimer's disease. The addition of progesterone or the administration of hormone replacement in the combined form as oestrogen and progesterone wipes out any protection that could be gained by using oestrogen only. There are numerous oestrogen receptors in the brain in the area responsible for cognition.

- Some believe that oestrogen deficiency is associated with Alzheimer's disease.

- Both Tau bodies and amyloid plaques are reduced in the presence of oestrogen and allows oestrogen deficiency to be considered as a risk factor for developing Alzheimer's disease.

Notes

Notes

_____

_____

_____

_____

_____

_____

_____

_____

_____

_____

_____

_____

_____

_____

_____

_____

_____

_____

_____

_____

_____

Chapter 9
Effects of Head Trauma

- Common causes of head trauma

- What does the science tell us?

- The role of vitamins

- Pause For Thought

- Take Home Nuggets

- Pages for personal notes

Reclining in the comfort of the armchairs and sofas which are acceptable elements of furnishings in our modern homes, we claim to entertain ourselves with the emotional cheers evoked by many contact sports, as we support the victors and try to explain why their opponents have lost. We have seen boxers repeatedly enter the fight ring walking with great fanfare and splendour yet leave the boxing ring on stretchers; we have seen players of American football carried off the playing field on stretchers unconscious, yet we in these modern times continue to support and cheer these sports on. We have not, even in these modern times, seriously considered how best we can protect participants in these events from themselves. Instead, we seem happier as if to pick up the pieces, as opposed to developing preventative strategies: we seem more interested in addressing the resultant morbidity.

Among the clearest instance of this morbidity in recent memory points to the sad deterioration of the boxer, Mohammad Ali, the self-proclaimed greatest of all time, a claim which many will not argue with but the purist will almost universally admit that he allowed himself to absorb too much punishment in the ring. Somewhere I read that this practice was on at least one occasion employed to get his opponent tired before he knocked him out. In the end, though, this previously talkative, bouncy, mobile athlete appeared to be a mere shell of his younger years as he struggled with the ill effects of Parkinson's disease, a condition which folks are eager to associate with his years in the ring. Whether you agree or not, the slurred speech and disjointed movements of many a previous fighter lend credence to this position. Many an American national football player has been diagnosed with chronic traumatic encephalopathy (CTE) and traumatic brain injury (TBI) posthumously. So, this finding combined with the pitiful sight of the shuffling gait and struggles of the one-time loquacious champion boxer serves to keep this issue in our conversations.

What does the science tell us?

- Traumatic brain injury is now known to be a leading cause of a condition called chronic traumatic encephalopathy (CTE), a progressive neurological disease that is believed to have been caused by trauma to the head earlier in life. CTE is now also known to mimic Parkinson's disease, Alzheimer's and other neurodegenerative diseases, leading to a shrinkage of the brain. At the molecular level there are many similarities between CTE and brain illnesses such as Parkinson's disease, Alzheimer's disease, and other neurodegenerative diseases.

- The similarities include a chronic inflammation of the brain, leading to disruption of the intercellular and intracellular messengers.

- There is also damage to the glucose metabolism in the nervous system, leading to suboptimal levels of energy, since the brain is dependent on glucose as its main energy source.

- Interference and possibly disruption of the circulation of the cerebrospinal fluid which washes the brain and its cells, critical to clearing toxins from the brain. Thus, although the immediate trauma to the head may cause some concern, there is a more sinister long-term sequel which raises its head in later life with ominous features. Is there anything that we can do to salvage the situation, short of placing a ban on all contact sports, I hear you ask?

In our searches we have come up with useful titbits which can protect us against this problem. We have found neuro-prophylactic compounds which can function in the prevention of the results of concussion, several years, even decades, after the initial insult.

A meta-analysis of published studies on the issue about the neuro-prophylactic compounds reveals that many of these compounds are antioxidants. This may not be surprising, recognising that there is an inflammatory and oxidative component to CTE.

Resveratrol, a flavonoid, is one such compound. While we await the results of human studies, multiple in vitro and animal studies have shown it is able to cross the blood-brain barrier and leads to the improvement in symptoms that develop from TBI (stroke and spinal cord injury).

Animal studies further suggest that resveratrol can improve both behaviour and neurological activity when it is given following head trauma. It has also been shown to slow the progression of neurodegenerative diseases like Alzheimer's.

It is believed that resveratrol can reduce intracerebral pressure by reducing brain oedema, and it can be used to treat anxiety, and improve functional performance and memory, whilst simultaneously enhancing movement.

It is believed that resveratrol can have these effects on the neuronal system because of its anti-inflammatory activity. Green tea has also been shown to have remarkable neuroprotective effect.

Green tea has at least three components which are known to be neuroprotective:

- Epigallocatechin-3-gallate (EGCG) is a flavonoid like resveratrol. It can cross the blood-brain barrier and enter the brain where it has been shown to improve cognitive function after neurological trauma. In animal studies it has been shown to be protective in Amyotrophic lateral sclerosis (ALS), Parkinson disease (PD) and Alzheimer's Disease (AD).

- L-theanine is a unique amino acid that is thought to give green tea its relaxing qualities. Like EGCG, it has been shown to be anti-inflammatory to nerve tissue and to protect it from injury.

- Methylxanthine, also known as caffeine, works as a non-selective adenosine receptor antagonist. This allows it to model and modify cell signals in the nerves, as well as to enhance healing after injury. Caffeine intake has been shown in numerous studies to be neuroprotective, and to decrease intracranial swelling as well as inflammation. An interesting observational study showed a 22% reduction in Parkinson's disease with coffee, and a 28% reduction with tea. Adenosine levels, which are affected by caffeine, are elevated following TBI. The elevated caffeine levels in cerebrospinal fluid is associated with improved outcome of TBI. This we believe results from caffeine ingestion and so we encourage increased caffeine intake.

Baicalin is another flavonoid obtained from Chinese skullcap which has a long history of use for hysteria, nervous tension, epilepsy and chorea. It has been studied extensively for its use in brain disorders.

The role of vitamins

Vitamin E has been shown in several studies to be effective in protecting the brain from the damage of injury. The high anti-oxidant activity of vitamin E can sometimes result in altering the vitamin E itself, leading to increased oxidation. To reduce that possibility, it is usual practice to give vitamin E with vitamin C simultaneously.

In addition to vitamin C and E, vitamin D acts like a hormone and seems to enhance the positive effects of progesterone.

Creatinine, an amino acid, is useful in maintaining proper brain and muscle function. TBI lowers the creatinine levels in the brain, and giving creatinine to animals lessens the amount of brain damage caused by subsequent injury. Creatinine may also be involved in improving metabolism and energy in tissues, including brain tissue. In patients following TBI, creatinine is believed to be involved in protecting the brain from damage which leads to better function, including cognitive function and behaviour than in individuals not receiving the supplements.

Pause For Thought

- Can contact sport cause brain injury?
- What is TBI?
- What is CTE?
- Could this have been a contributing factor to the great Mohammed Ali slurred speech?
- What is the similarity between TBI, Alzheimer's and Parkinson's disease?
- Does CTE lead to a disruption of the brain's glucose metabolism and its ability to cleanse itself?
- Can we protect ourselves from this condition of CTE?

Take Home Nuggets

- At the molecular level, TBI, CTE, Alzheimer's disease, Parkinson's all have a similar underlying association with oxidation and inflammation.

- There are many compounds which fall into the group of neuroprophylactic compounds which have shown some promise in reducing the impact of trauma in causing Chronic Traumatic Encephalopathy (CTE), and they are all antioxidants. This lends credence to the role of oxidation in these neurological conditions.

Notes

_____

_____

_____

_____

_____

_____

_____

_____

_____

_____

_____

_____

_____

_____

_____

_____

_____

_____

_____

_____

Notes

Chapter 10
Synopsis

- The devastation of the disease

- Tenets of root causes

- Infective agents

- Oxygen starvation

- Sleep deprivation

- Head trauma

- Heavy metals

- Pause For Thought

- Take Home Nuggets

- Pages for personal notes

The diagnosis of a fatal disease is devastating news to the recipient and carers, but to me a loved one slowly descending into a memoryless shell of their former self is not only pitiful to observe, but also emotionally draining to family, friends and carers. This is made even less palatable with the recognition that conventional medicine has had little or no success in the management of this condition after over a century since it was first identified. Clinically and realistically, therefore, the diagnosis of Alzheimer's disease is a sentence of a prolonged agonising death, a gradual process which may last between 3 and 11 years, during which time you are almost forced to recognise your relative, your associate's journey on his/her daily decline with hardly any bright moments or days. So traumatic and draining is this experience, not only physically but also emotionally, and financially as well, and invasive to the family dynamics that one is willing to cast a blind eye to the pursuance of a semblance of some dignity in the search for clinics such as Dignitas, which is yet to be globally accepted as an appropriate manner to minimise, reduce or curtail the pain that this illness inevitably brings.

To many, Alzheimer's disease represents the harshest of diagnosis made to our elderly parents and relatives. This may be so because not only is the disease without a cure using traditional medicines, but it is also progressive; our relatives appear as mere shells; they do not seem physically unwell, they just have a dysfunctional brain. They therefore navigate the world without much insight into their activity. You may hasten to say that this is normal since we all do so at various times for differing periods. The difference, though, is that the actions of our loved ones seem to be an act of deliberate helplessness. They seem to be a mere shell driven by a state of social irresponsibility to conduct acts that we may consider wholly socially reprehensible and for which they seem to show no remorse and may even argue that theirs was the right thing to do. In our cultured environments, we are driven to attempt to chastise, to try to correct our seniors for their unsavoury behaviour. This on occasions leads to the abuse of the elderly. None of us, I dare say, would feel comfortable abusing our parents. With that in mind, is it more humane to take them to the Dignitas clinic for a dignified farewell, or is it more appropriate to watch their continuous mental decline before our very eyes? On the one hand, we may feel the guilt and shame of being responsible for our relatives' demise, a mental strain with which we must continue to live versus the heartlessness of being unable to assist loved ones as they continue to decline towards the abyss of depleted mentation. Neither of which is an appropriate choice, I hear you say.

It is because of this dilemma that there is a need for a closer look at this disease process to try to understand its root cause. Much work has been done and is still ongoing, resulting in a continuous upgrade of our understanding of this disease process. Our understanding as reflected in the text of this manuscript encourages hope for the future as we explore the current understanding about the root cause of this disease.

Tenets of root cause(s)

Our current knowledge strongly hints at a multifactorial basis for this disease. Among the commonly accepted causative agents are: (a) infective agents; (b) oxygen starvation, particularly at night during our sleep; (c) sleep deprivation; (d) head trauma; and (e) heavy metals and their toxic effects.

Infective agents

The focus here is on the role played by herpes simplex virus type 1. This virus seems to be the major culprit in the occurrence of cold sores which tend to manifest themselves as lesions around the mouth. These viruses are ubiquitous and may affect an individual even if he/she is unaware of having the virus. The virus can be passed on to other individuals by kissing, sharing eating utensils etc. These viruses have the ability to lie dormant for extended periods, only manifesting their presence during times of immunosuppression. It is felt that during these periods of dormancy, the viruses tend to live in the neuronal system. If that be the case and recognising the focus of their attack, it is very possible that they can make the relatively short trip from the mouth and facial areas to the brain where they can have harmful effects. Though this may seem an assumption, it is known that viruses such as varicella, which causes chickenpox, can live in the nervous system for years before manifesting along nerve roots with a burning, painful, discoloured lesion referred to as shingles. Varicella is a type of herpes virus, so it has the capacity to behave similarly. Furthermore, there are several scientific publications in world literature which document the presence of herpes simplex type 1 antibodies in juxtaposition with brain lesions commonly associated with Alzheimer's disease. If viral infection was the only known cause of Alzheimer's disease, then treating this condition would be focussed on halting the proliferation of the virus, followed by optimising our immunisation so that our bodies would be able to clear these viruses, but other factors such as oxygen starvation seem to be culpable.

Oxygen starvation

The major energy source for the brain is glucose. As a source of energy, glucose must be metabolised. There are two plausible pathways: anaerobic and aerobic respiration. Anaerobic respiration, though, is a very wasteful process, which produces only a net gain of 5.5% of the energy produced by aerobic respiration; so, you will agree that this would not be a first- choice option for the brain in getting its energy requirement. The preferred pathway would be aerobic respiration, for which oxygen is required. Any factor which reduces the oxygen supply to the brain interferes with its function and may cause it to have long-term far-reaching dysfunctional results. As an obstetrician, one of the areas we are trained to explore is any suggestion of oxygen deprivation to the foetus in a patient. So important is oxygen supply to the brain that even being deprived of oxygen during intrauterine life or during birth can adversely affect the baby. We see evidence of deprivation of oxygen in babies who are born whether vaginally or by Caesarean section, though more common during vaginal births, in the form of various neurological manifestations such as quadriplegia or its other cousins. We have also seen that in adults who have had a multiplicity of strokes, impaired vascular circulation, diabetes, cardiac disease and high blood pressure issues there is an increased tendency to develop neurological challenges such as Alzheimer's later in life. It is for this reason, among others, that if you suffer from apnoea (excessive snoring) you should see your general practitioner who could, among other things, recommend fitting you with a CPAP machine which essentially forces air into your lungs. Apart from the possibility of oxygen starvation, which may happen during sleep, how else can sleep help to ensure brain health, and halt and possibly reverse a debilitating neurodegenerative disease such as Alzheimer's?

Sleep deprivation

Research tells us that the brain is constantly cleaning itself, getting rid of various toxins to which it inadvertently becomes exposed – for example, heavy metals. The cleansing activity of the brain is conducted by specialised cells which are carried around in the brain by cerebrospinal fluid. These cells cleanse the surface of the brain during the day because the brain is so actively involved in other activities that only a small fraction of the energy expended during the day is used for cleaning purposes. These specialised cells are called glial cells. At night during sleep the brain is less active in directing our life activities and can spend a greater proportion of its energy in cleaning itself. There are two important factors which occur during sleep which facilitate and optimise the brain activity to cleanse itself. The brain physiologically shrinks: this has the effect of functionally increasing the size of the ducts in the brain, allowing more space for the cerebrospinal fluid to course through the brain, and this brings the brain cells closer to the cerebrospinal fluid, making for more efficient cellular cleaning. Secondly, the energy utilisation in the brain increases 20-fold: the increased need and use of energy indicate the effectiveness and importance of the cleansing mechanism. Compared to being awake, there is indirect evidence If we do not obtain sufficient sleep, then the cleansing of the brain would be compromised and so incomplete, leaving behind toxins which will eventually accrue to cause long-term degenerative havoc on the brain. It is obvious that the less sleep one gets, the less efficient the brain will be at cleaning itself. Acquisition of seven to eight hours of sleep nightly is considered essential for adequate cleansing of the brain.

Head trauma

We have come to learn that repeat trauma to the head leads to a condition called traumatic brain injury, which leads to a condition called chronic traumatic encephalopathy (CTE), a progressive neurological disease that results from head trauma earlier in life. This CTE can mimic Parkinson's disease, Alzheimer's and other neurodegenerative diseases. In this case the brain literally shrinks: this is distinct from the physiological shrinkage of the brain during sleep. In this scenario, shrinkage because of previous head trauma leading to CTE, there are a number of similarities with other known degenerative neurological conditions. There are also anatomical changes which take place in the brain of one so afflicted. There is evidence of chronic inflammation in the brain which leads to disruption of intracellular and intercellular messengers. There is damage to the glucose metabolism in the nervous system which leads to suboptimal energy production. There is also a disruption in the cerebrospinal fluid circulation, a continuous circulation of the cerebrospinal fluid which is essential for brain cleansing. Fortunately, with time we are becoming increasingly aware of neuroprophylactic compounds that can be used to prevent the long-term sequelae of CTE. Compounds like resveratrol, green tea and even caffeine have found some utility in this area. Lastly, we talk about the impact of heavy metals on our brain health.

Heavy metals

In society we are continuously exposed to a barrage of heavy metals. These are inhaled and ingested for the most part. These heavy metals include aluminium, copper and mercury, which are virtually ubiquitous. These enter our bodies through various modalities in our drinks, in our foods, in our oral care hygiene, skin care etc. Since these heavy metals are so common it is difficult to avoid them, and it would therefore be more sensible to try to develop mechanisms by which we can avoid them from impacting our health. To our rescue comes the practice of chelation, a means by which these heavy metals are bound and excreted from our bodies. Until recently this was an expensive undertaking requiring intravenous administration, but more recently it has also been offered as an oral preparation which is much more user-friendly.

Additionally, there are numerous drugs in common use which are associated with the occurrence of Alzheimer's.

We talk of oxybutynin, a drug commonly used for the treatment of an overactive bladder; acetazolamide (Diamox), used to treat glaucoma, epilepsy, altitude sickness, periodic paralysis, idiopathic intracranial hypertension and heart failure, and to change the pH of urine; carbamazepine (Tegretol), used to treat epilepsy and nerve pain; gabapentin (Neurontin), used to treat epilepsy and nerve pain; lamotrigine (Lamictal), used to treat partial seizures, primary generalized tonic-clonic seizures, bipolar disorder maintenance and Lennox-Gastaut syndrome, bipolar depression, fibromyalgia, schizophrenia and unipolar depression; levetiracetam (Keppra), used to treat epilepsy; oxcarbazepine (Trileptal), used to treat certain types of seizures in adults and children 6 years of age and older; pregabalin (Lyrica), used to treat epilepsy, anxiety and nerve pain; rufinamide (Banzel), used in conjunction with other medications to control seizure in people who have Lennox-Gastaut syndrome; topiramate (Topamax), used to treat epilepsy, and prevent migraine, thought to work by reducing bursts of electrical activity in the brain and restoring the normal balance of nerve activity; valproic acid (Depakote), used to treat epilepsy, bipolar disorder and migraine; and zonisamide (Zonegran), used to treat symptoms of epilepsy and Parkinson's disease. It is quite interesting to note that the bulk of drugs known to be associated with the occurrence of Alzheimer's are used to treat brain/neurological disorders.

Pause For Thought

- Why could Alzheimer's disease be considered the most devastating disease known to man?
- Does Alzheimer's disease have a single cause?
- Are we able to protect ourselves from this ominous condition?
- Do antioxidants have a role to play?
- Is brain Shrinkage a factor in many neurodegenerative diseases?

Take Home Nuggets

- Alzheimer's disease may be considered as the most devastating disease of our time, since we see our loved ones progressively die with us being unwilling spectators. Death can be described as the absence of a heartbeat, but if the brain is dead, you are for all intents and purposes also dead. With Alzheimer's disease and its multifactorial causes, the process is the same, progressive reduction and shrinkage of brain tissue, because of the death of portions of the brain. This reflects a very sad and emotionally draining state.

- Though with a disease such as cancer, the patient may be dying but he/she may retain their wits, can still laugh and play with children and grandchildren in Alzheimer's, the patient quickly becomes the child by his/her progressive loss of the features considered necessary to be an adult.

- We at Philburn Academy believe that we cannot just simply talk about it, but we must aim did at the beginning of this discussion of Alzheimer's disease but we must aim to do all that we can to safeguard ourselves against this ominous condition.

Notes

Notes

Epilogue

Reclaiming your health is not only possible but necessary if you want to add years to your life and life to your years. Let us explore how this is possible. We look at the 9 most common chronic health issues of today and indicate how these can be overcome. We will explore the disease process, trying to understand their causation, and determine through reliable scientific research how to keep these health challenges at bay. We will also delve into common-sense practices which will play invaluable roles in rendering the disease dormant and in some cases completely reverse the disease process. We encourage the employment of various common-sense measures, as well as provide evidence on how the advised measures work. We are strong proponents of social and preventative medicine and recognise the failure of traditional approaches in the fight against a variety of disease processes.

In this series of 12 books, we will produce easy-to-read manuscripts about each of the nine most common chronic medical conditions, and a book on women's health after the menopause, as well as a book on men's health in which we will question the issue of andropause and address some of the challenges of getting more advanced in age.

With experience and training in organic chemistry, biochemistry and medicine, both as a clinical practitioner and as a trainer for in excess of 30 years, coupled with my years of teaching, I believe that I am uniquely positioned to help you add years to your life and life to your years by attacking and overcoming the vices of modern living which have almost succeeded in overcoming and burdening our very existence through these nine most common chronic ailments. The last three books in this series not only address the issues of getting older, but also suggest methods which you can employ to present the most active versions of yourself even in your twilight years. The final book in this series was empowered by my stem cell research, the legal and ethical issues, during the preparation and fulfilment for the master's degree in law which I was able to complete.

Notes

_____

_____

_____

_____

_____

_____

_____

_____

_____

_____

_____

_____

_____

_____

_____

_____

_____

_____

_____

_____

_____

_____

Notes

_____

_____

_____

_____

_____

_____

_____

_____

_____

_____

_____

_____

_____

_____

_____

_____

_____

_____

_____

_____

_____

www.ingramcontent.com/pod-product-compliance
Lightning Source LLC
Chambersburg PA
CBHW081819200326
41597CB00023B/4309